A Thai Herbal

D1375999

A Thai Herbal

Traditional Recipes for

Health and Harmony

C. Pierce Salguero

FINDHORN
Press

© C. Pierce Salguero 2003

First published in 2003

ISBN 1-84409-004-3

All rights reserved.
The contents of this book may not be reproduced in any form,
except for short extracts for quotation or review,
without the written permission of the publisher.

British Library Cataloguing-in-Publication Data.
A catalogue record for this book is available from the British Library.

Edited by Lynn Barton
Layout by Pam Bochel
Illustrations by David Schuster
Cover design by Thierry Bogliolo

Printed and bound by WS Bookwell, Finland

Published by

Findhorn Press

305a The Park, Findhorn
Forres IV36 3TE
Scotland
Tel 01309 690582
Fax 01309 690036

e-mail: info@findhornpress.com
findhornpress.com

OM NAMO SHIVAGO SIRASA AHANG KARUNIKO
SAPASATANANG OSATA TIPAMANTANG
PAPASO SURIYAJANTANG KOMARAPATO PAGASESI WANTAMI
BANDITO SUMETASO A-LOKA SUMANAHOMI

PIYO-TEWA MANUSANANG PIYO-PROMA NAMUTAMO
PIYO-NAKA SUPANANANG PINISRIYONG NAMAMIHANG
NAMOPUTAYA NAVON-NAVEAN NASATIT-NASATEAN
A-HIMAMA NAVEAN-NAVE NAPITANG-VEAN NAVEANMAHAKO
A-HIMAMA PIYONGMAMA NAMOPUTAYA

NA-A NAVA LOKA PAYATI WINASANTI

We invite the spirit of our founder,
the Father Doctor "Shivago," who taught us
through his saintly life.
Please bring to us knowledge of nature,
and show us the true medicine in the universe.
Through this prayer, we request your help,
that through our hands,
you will bring wholeness and health to the body of our client.

The god of healing dwells in the heavens high
while mankind remains in the world below.
In the name of the founder, may the heavens
be reflected in the earth,
so that this healing medicine may encircle the world.

We pray for the one whom we touch,
that he will be happy
and that any illness will be released from him.

This book is dedicated to my wife, Marcie,

whose countless cups of tea kept me going

through my writings in Thailand.

Table of Contents

Acknowledgements

The main source of information for this collection were my teachers and contacts in Chiang Mai. I am especially indebted to the staff at the Shivagakomarpaj Traditional Medicine Hospital for allowing me access to their herbal course text books, and to Pikun and Maew, both at Lek Chaiya Massage for helping with the translation and augmentation of this material. I have utmost gratitude to my massage teachers, including Daeng, Pramost, and "Mama" Lek among others, for sparking my interest in holistic medicine, and for helping me to come to a fuller understanding of Thai culture. My thanks is also due to Chef Somphon, Welcome to Chiang Mai Chiang Rai, the RDI, and Chongkol Setthakorn, who have generously allowed me to use their material in these pages.

Introduction

Traditional Thai medicine—a combination of yoga, acupressure, herbal therapy, and dietary regimens—is a colorful art form that reflects Thailand's wide range of cultural influences. A holistic system of traditional medicine practiced in Thai villages and royal courts for millennia, it continues to grow and evolve to this day.

The healing systems of Southeast Asia (including Thailand) have been studied by ethnobotanists and anthropologists for decades, but only recently have Western holistic health practitioners taken an interest in learning more about these rich traditions. We are realizing that the traditional medicine of China and India—although the most popular—are not the only vibrant healing traditions in Asia. The analysis of new medical systems is a vital field of study, a crucial addition to the world's stock of medical knowledge, and a breath of the fresh air of ancient wisdom in the modern age.

Thai medicine, like most of the Eastern medical traditions, is not only about curing disease; it is about taking control of one's health, promoting wellness, and improving quality of life. In Thailand, herbs are a part of a holistic system of wellness that takes into account the whole self—mind, body, and spirit—and puts medical knowledge into the hands of the patient. Thai medicine teaches us that with appropriate understanding of herbs, we can learn to live in harmony with the changing seasons and the changes in our lives. With a handful of medicinal plants, we can successfully treat the most common ailments we are likely to encounter in daily life. With herbal tonics, we can strengthen our bodies and immune systems in order to prevent disease in the first place. With traditional recipes, we can lessen the toxic effects of pollution and pesticides we ingest, enhance our energy levels, immunity, and sexuality, and increase our longevity and happiness.

This collection is the product of my research in Bangkok and Chiang Mai, Northern Thailand, over a period from 1997 to 2001. I have arrived at the latest incarnation of this collection by analyzing over 150 herbs, determining how they are used by traditional Thai healers and how they are regarded by other systems such as Western, Ayurvedic, and Chinese herbalism. (My sources for these comparisons are listed in the bibliography.) This collection is a large and informative compendium of the medicinal herbs used in Thailand, but I have taken much care to ensure that it is a readable and practical guide for beginning and professional herbalists alike. I have attempted to translate traditional ideas into a modern context, hoping to bring this ancient wisdom into the realm of daily life. Most of all, I have tried to make the subject of traditional medicine fun, offering easy recipes for remedies, cosmetics, and cuisine that will make the world of Thai tradition come alive in our homes.

Many of the therapeutic herbs in this collection have been used in Chinese, Ayurvedic, or Western herbalism, and are available to modern herbalists and patients in the grocery store or herbalist shop. Sometimes, however, there is no correspondence. Some of the herbs in this collection are difficult to procure in the West, and several have no common names other than in the Thai language. Sometimes, the name exists, but the herbs remain far outside the scope of the familiar traditions. This, for me, is the most fascinating part of this endeavor. I believe that many treasures of traditional medicine still lie unknown. The medical systems of Southeast Asia are ancient repositories of healing wisdom, but they remain largely unstudied in comparison with other Asian traditions. What medicinal gems may be growing undiscovered in the mountain villages of Thailand? What secrets may the old-growth rainforests of Southeast Asia reveal? The process of discovery has only begun, and I hope that this collection encourages professional and amateur herbalists alike to experiment with new vistas.

C. Pierce Salguero
November 21, 2002
Charlottesville, Virginia

Chapter I

The Tradition of Thai Medicine

HISTORY OF THAI MEDICINE

Thai medicine, like most aspects of culture in Thailand, is based on indigenous tradition and a colorful blend of Indian, Chinese, and Khmer influences. The historical progenitor of Thai medicine, Jivaka Kumar Bhaccha (pronounced by Thais as "Shivago Komarpaj") is revered by almost all practitioners as the "Father Doctor" of Thai medicine. Jivaka was an historical figure, a contemporary of the Buddha, and personal physician to the Buddha's order of monks and nuns over 2,500 years ago. He was a renowned Ayurvedic doctor in his time and is considered by Thais to be the original teacher of the Thai massage system, as well as the source of Thailand's complex herb and mineral pharmacopoeia.

The Father Doctor plays a central role in the spiritual beliefs of Thai healers to this day. Most herbalists, masseurs, and traditional doctors maintain a shrine which includes statuettes of the Buddha and the Father Doctor side-by-side, and prayers such as the one at the beginning of this book are chanted daily to invoke the spirit of the Father Doctor to assist in the healing of patients.

Legends aside, however, it is difficult to tell how much of the Thai medical traditions actually came from the Ayurvedic masters. Ayurvedic ideas are mentioned frequently in the herbal texts of Thailand. However, it is not exactly clear how pervasive this influence is or at what point Indian ideas entered the Thai culture. What amount of influence came to Thailand from India, what amount came from other sources, and what was indigenous to Thailand is impossible to gauge, as there has been much overlap and cross-cultural exchange over the centuries.

According to Harald "Asokananda" Brust, the foremost Western writer on Thai massage, the historical origins of Thai Medicine are shrouded in mystery:

> *Despite what is known about Kumar Bhaccha, much of the origins of Thai massage and traditional Thai medicine still remain obscure. It is believed that the teachings of Kumar Bhaccha reached what is now Thailand at the same time as Buddhism—as early as the 3rd or 2nd century BC. It is unknown whether there was any indigenous form of [medicine] in the region before that time. Equally unknown is to what extent Chinese concepts of acupuncture and acupressure (as well as other aspects of traditional medicine) had any theoretical and practical influence... Nowadays it is impossible to definitively answer such questions, since for centuries medical knowledge was transmitted almost entirely orally from teacher to student following a teaching tradition also common in India.*[1]

Many parallels to Ayurveda can be found in the Thai tradition, and some Thai concepts (such as *tridosha* and *nadis*) even share the same names as their Ayurvedic counterparts. However, most scholars tend to think that these are later additions, rather than fundamentals of the Thai system. Jean Mulholland, one of the foremost anthropologists of Thai medicine, states in a discussion of one of the traditional herbal manuals:

> *I can no longer assert that Thai traditional medicine is based primarily on the philosophy of Ayurveda. Rather... the few short passages and recipes based on Ayurveda which do occur seem to have been superimposed at the beginning or end of sections of an already established text.*[2]

Viggo Brun and Trond Schumacher conclude that in the Thai system,

> *the theory [of Ayurveda]... is imported from India, is not integrated with practice, and functions only as a frame of reference or explanatory model.*[3]

Most experts on Thai medicine have likewise concluded that references to Ayurveda are not central to Thai herbalism. With this in mind, throughout this book I will only briefly touch upon Ayurveda as it applies to Thai herbalism. (Readers seeking more information should consult Dr. David Frawley's excellent book on Ayurvedic herbs listed in

---

[1] Asokananda (Harald Brust), *Thai Traditional Massage* (Bangkok: Editions Duang Kamol, 1990), 4–5.

[2] Jean Mulholland, "Ayurveda, Congenital Disease and Birthdays in Thai Traditional Medicine," <u>Journal of the Siam Society</u> 76 (1988): 175.

[3] Viggo Brun and Trond Schumacher, *Traditional Herbal Medicine in Northern Thailand* (Bangkok: White Lotus, 1994), 32.

the bibliography.) I will instead take the Thai tradition on its own terms and will concentrate on topics which have barely been covered by other authors: the indigenous philosophy and practice central to this fascinating system of healing.

THE TWO TRADITIONS

Scholars of Thai medicine have distinguished between the rural and the royal traditions, treating these two as distinct medical systems. There is much overlap between the two, as they share some terminology and herbal recipes. However, it is only the royal tradition that developed a formal theory of disease, symptoms, and treatment.

The Rural and Hill-Tribe Traditions

The rural and Hill-Tribe traditions tend to be informal, varying considerably from village to village, tribe to tribe, and indeed from practitioner to practitioner. The livelihood of the rural tradition lies in the hands of local male practitioners, famous in small circles for their healing "powers." Rural Thai and Hill-Tribe healers rarely attain the high levels of education that are prerequisite in the royal tradition. The medical knowledge is transmitted largely orally and through secret herbal manuscripts handed down from teacher to pupil. Whereas the royal medical practices have, in the past centuries, emphasized formal scientific treatises, rural Thai medicine has remained to this day more unorganized than centralized, more artistic than dogmatic, and more spiritual than scientific.

Because of the lack of formalized instruction, the local differences in practice, the language barrier, and the aura of secrecy which surrounds the tradition, rural herbal knowledge is difficult to collect, and even more difficult to study comprehensively. True to their secretive tradition, the herbal masters are not likely to give direct answers to theoretical questions and will sometimes intentionally mislead anthropologists looking to study their healing systems. While this may be frustrating to the modern scientific mind, it is important to realize that some of the most important practices in the rural tradition are difficult or impossible to explain verbally. Much of the rural and Hill-Tribe practice remains shrouded in spiritual tradition and is difficult to translate to a modern context. Many of these healers are more properly shamans and utilize a broad range of shamanic techniques such as exorcisms, amulet charming, and incantations of magic formulas.

It is not my intention to focus on the village traditions in this work. To my knowledge, there are no schools in Thailand that offer courses in rural medicine, and it is exceedingly difficult for Westerners to study under individual practitioners. To this day, there has not been very much written on the subject by either Thai or Western researchers. Of the few that have been written, one eloquent and interesting study (Brun and Schumacher, *Traditional Medicine in Northern Thailand*) is mentioned in the bibliography at the end of this book as an excellent introduction to this complicated field.

The Wat Po School of Royal Medicine

At the same time that more informal traditions persisted for centuries in the countryside, temples and hospitals under royal patronage were establishing a consistent system of medical theory and practice. The royal tradition was based on traditional rural lore but became organized and codified with the introduction of Ayurvedic and Western concepts. Buddhism, and along with it many Indian ideas, arrived in the kingdom of Siam in several waves throughout antiquity. A constant flow of information came to the region along with Chinese, Arab, and Indian merchants. European explorers arrived as early as 1504. The medical tradition picked up something from each of these groups as they came through.

According to Somchintana Ratarasarn, a traditional medicine researcher,

> by about 1600 AD the secular medical system of the Thai people had been established, and had attained maturity as a coherent and highly effective system of health care. It was sustained by... the king, his appointed officials, and the intellectual elite.[4]

The Wat Po temple was established in the late 1700s under the founder of the current Thai dynasty, Rama I. In 1836, Rama III ordered an extensive renovation of the grounds. At that time, 60 inscribed stone tablets bearing acupressure charts and 1100 herbal recipes were placed in the walls of the temple to preserve medical knowledge for future generations. Over 80 statues depicting massage techniques and yoga postures were erected throughout the grounds as well. These statues and stone tablets can still be seen by visitors to the temple today, and they still form the basis of the royal school of Thai medicine.

From 1895 to 1907, Wat Po's Traditional Medical School published several important herbal manuals to disseminate this valuable information throughout Thailand. These texts are a summary of the ancient traditional lore preserved at Wat Po and are a useful font of information for Thai and Western scholars. Furthermore, these texts

---

4 Somchintana Ratarasarn, *The Principles and Concepts of Thai Classical Medicine* (Bangkok: Thai Khadi Research Institute, Thammasat University, 1986), 277–78.

provide the basic curriculum for the school of traditional medicine that still operates on the grounds of the temple.

Unfortunately, to this day, the Wat Po manuals have not appeared in complete English translation. While tourists are able to take short courses on Thai massage in English, the herbalism classes are limited to the Thai language, and therefore remain relatively inaccessible to Westerners. However, enough information has become available to provide a clear picture of the medical practices of the royal school. The theories discussed in this book are based mainly on this royal tradition of Wat Po. Information that comes specifically from the Wat Po texts is noted, as is information that more properly pertains to the rural and Hill-Tribe traditions.

THE CIRCLE OF LIFE

Before embarking on an explanation of the details of Thai herbalism in specific, it would be useful to summarize a few concepts central to Thai medicine as a whole. In Thai philosophy, human life is holistically viewed as a combination of three essences:

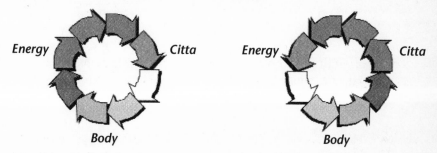

Energy   Citta   Energy   Citta

Body   Body

In this Circle of Life, there is a constant flow between the three essences. **Body** refers to the substance of which we are made, the combination of atoms that make up our physical self. The Thai word *citta*, translated usually as **mind/heart**, is understood to be the entire non-physical human being—all of our thoughts, emotions, and spirit that makes up our inner lives, or our inner self. Being rooted in Buddhism, which does not recognize the existence of a soul, Thai philosophy states that the *citta* is a part of our being, not a separate entity, but tied to the physical body. **Energy**, in the Thai system, holds mind, heart and body together. Analogous to the Chinese idea of *qi* (or *chi*) and to the Indian concept of *prana*, this energy is an intangible flow that courses through the body via specific meridians called *nadis*. As in the Indian system, the Thai model recognizes 72,000 of these *nadis*, running throughout the body, which do not have anatomical counterparts but which are well known to traditional healers.

The Thai tradition recognizes diseases caused by germs, allergies, environmental factors, heredity, and emotional or psychological imbalance. However, in the Thai system, the root cause of any and all disease is the imbalance of the body, *citta,* and energy. When the three essences are balanced, the human organism enjoys health and well-being. The imbalance of the three essences causes this natural health and immunity to break down, leaving the organism vulnerable to disease.

Acute injuries such as falling and breaking a bone, or those received in a car accident, would seem to be exceptions to this rule, but many Thai healers claim to be able to perceive these events on the energetic level before they manifest on the physical plane. Nevertheless, the links between the essences are often not hard to see. It is clear that even a purely physical disorder can soon negatively affect the mind, emotions, and energy, as physical stagnation and trauma can lead to depression, anxiety, fatigue, and low immunity. Likewise, excessive or depleted energy will cause the body and *citta* to become imbalanced, and imbalance of the mind and/or emotions causes energetic and physical strain. All three essences are interconnected and mutually affect each other continuously throughout life.

An understanding of the Circle of Life idea leads Thai medicine, like all holistic systems, to approach disease not as a merely physical phenomenon, but as simultaneously a mental, physical, and energetic problem. Thus, in the Thai tradition, all ailments are treated holistically. All parts of the circle are interconnected. Maintaining balance of the three essences is therefore the primary focus of traditional Thai medicine.

THE BRANCHES OF THAI MEDICINE

Traditional medicine in Thailand is historically split into three disciplines: religious or spiritual healing, manipulative massage, and dietary regimens and herbal medicine. Each treats a different aspect of the Circle of Life.

Mind/Heart Therapy: Spiritual healing

Spiritual or magical treatment remains prevalent in modern Thailand, even within the relatively more scientific Royal Tradition. Thai medicine emphasizes the spiritual well-being of the patient and holds that many diseases flow from a troubled heart or mind. For this reason, even modern Thai healing is enveloped in a rich and intricate tradition of prayer, meditation, mantras, and mythology based around Buddhist and shamanic ideas, which are designed to heal the *citta* in order to heal the whole self.

In Thailand, spiritual healing often involves elaborate ceremonies that include the patient's family and friends in the healing process. While these rites may seem merely interesting and unusual to the Westerner, they are an important part of the healing arts in Thai culture and sometimes affect seemingly miraculous cures. Certain meditations, mantras, breathing techniques, and visualizations play a role in this process, as do magic incantations and healing amulets. More information on these techniques is presented in detail in my book, *The Spiritual Healing of Traditional Thailand.*

Energy Therapy: Thai Massage

Interestingly, Thai massage is not considered to be bodywork, but rather is seen in Thailand primarily a therapy of energy. Masseurs do not soothe muscles with stroking Swedish-massage-style movements, but rather apply acupressure to certain points on the body in order to increase the flow of energy through the *nadis* to relieve symptoms and stimulate healing. Linked by these energy circuits, the part of the body massaged may be entirely different from the part of the body injured. (For example, a massage to treat insomnia will concentrate mainly on the legs, and a massage to treat cough may focus on the arms and legs.) These techniques can only be understood by looking at where the *nadis* run within the body and which systems they affect. More information on Thai massage and energy meridian therapy is presented in my book, *The Encyclopedia of Traditional Thai Massage.*

While Thai massage has enjoyed increasing popularity in the West as of late, and there have been several books on the subject, it is a field that, in Thailand, remains intimately tied to the other three branches of traditional medicine. Part of the purpose of this series is to provide a framework of Thai medicine as a whole, through which Thai massage can be seen in a holistic context. (For more information on the use of herbs in massage, see *Chapter IV.*)

Body Therapy: Dietary Regimens and Herbal Medicine

This book is mainly concerned with dietary and herbal therapy. Herbs and food affect the human organism by causing physiological changes in body chemistry, and therefore these are considered to be primarily therapies for the body essence. But this does not mean that herbalism is limited to the physical body. Because of the intimate link between body, *citta,* and energy, by ingesting therapeutic herbs, minerals, and other natural substances, we can affect the healing process within the physical, mental, and energetic selves. These ideas are discussed in further detail in the next four chapters.

It should be noted that Thai herbalists typically use herbal medicine only as a last resort. Solutions to problems are usually sought from dietary regimens first, as the cause of most imbalances are to be found in what we are or are not eating. (An old Thai axiom states that the cause of disease is in the stomach.) When herbal medicines are prescribed, it is always in conjunction with dietary recommendations. By understanding the energetic properties of the foods we eat, we can learn to harmonize our diets with our own constitutions and our environment, in order to avoid future imbalances that lead to illness. A section on dietary regimens, or food medicine, is presented in *Chapter III.*

HOLISTIC HEALING

Although they tend to specialize in one area of treatment or another, traditional Thai healers would advocate the use of spiritual healing, massage, and dietary and herbal therapy in harmony to cure disease by holistically addressing body, mind, heart, and energy together. As an example, hepatitis may be treated by certain herbal teas and by avoiding foods that overstimulate the liver, by massage of the *nadis* associated with the liver, or by certain types of visualizations accompanied by life-style changes. Any of these therapies alone would work to some extent, but a holistic approach where all three therapies are undertaken in conjunction will prove to be much more effective.

In the Thai tradition, all ailments are treated holistically. Although it has been common to the East for centuries, and was common in the West in the times of the Ancient Greeks, the holistic treatment of body, mind, heart, and energy is an idea that is foreign to most Western physicians. Western, or allopathic, doctors tend to look only at the physical body, and are often ignorant of the mental and energetic aspects of disease. This purely physical approach may work well enough in the case of a broken arm or other bodily trauma, but it is notably less effective in treatment of chronic diseases such as cancer, diabetes, and heart disease, and disorders such as depression, chronic anxiety, and fibromyalgia. Holistic medicine follows a balanced approach to healing, treating the body, mind, heart, and energy together through a combination of therapies designed to strengthen the body's own defenses, instill a sense of mental and physical harmony, and cure these types of diseases from the root.

In modern times, there is often skepticism as to how the three essences are intertwined. Often, rural Thais profess many beliefs that would be deemed by most Westerners as contrary to logic. For example, miraculous cures are often attributed to the Buddha, to a particularly powerful monk, or to a pilgrimage site. Most Western doctors would not accept this as a valid explanation, but again, I prefer to view these instances in the light of the Circle of Life, as the intimate relationship of body, mind, heart, and energy.

Allopathic medicine has long recognized what researchers call the placebo effect, and have been stumped as to how sugar pills can affect a cure in patients with serious life-threatening diseases. The practitioner of Eastern medicine would not be surprised with these examples, as they are simply cases where the mind/heart was able to cure the physical body. Likewise, the clinical effectiveness of acupuncture has been regarded with much suspicion by Western doctors, who refuse to accept the notion of invisible energy meridians. Again, the Eastern practitioner would be completely at home with the idea of energy therapy curing the physical body.

If these therapies have not been explained to the satisfaction of the empirical scientist, this may be due to the fact that they have not yet been studied rigorously enough. But, for most traditional Thai practitioners, the question of how exactly the mind, heart, and energy affect the body is secondary to the practical reality that they *do*. A quote from the Buddhist scriptures illustrates this point:

> It is as if a man had been wounded by a poisoned arrow, and when attended by a physician, he were to say, "I will not allow you to remove this arrow until I have learned the caste, the age, the occupation, the birthplace, and the motivation of the person who wounded me." That man would die before having learned all this.

Quite possibly, the Circle of Life may never be "proven" by the medical establishment. But the bottom line is that holistic therapies work and should be used. These therapies have been shown to work over centuries of practice by Asian countries. At the very least, we can say that *citta*-therapies and energy-therapies stimulate the natural healing processes of the body, and therefore, they can assist with treatment of any and all diseases. And we can also say that quite often, holistic healing techniques seemingly work wonders where allopathic medicine has repeatedly failed.

TRADITIONAL THAI MEDICINE TODAY AND IN THE FUTURE

In recent years, holistic Asian treatments for mind, body, and energy have slowly begun to gain acceptance by the Western world. While Western medicine still emphasizes body treatments such as prescription drugs, surgery, and so on, alternative, or complementary, therapies have lately gained much respect in the eyes of the public, and even are begrudgingly accepted in some medical circles. Techniques such as acupuncture and massage have become part of the modern hospital setting in many places, often even being covered under insurance plans.

As East and West each become more familiar with the wisdom of the other, it is natural that the best of the ancient and the modern will come together in a new synthesis. It is the challenge of the modern era to create this new model of medicine, and this model will begin with a deeper understanding of the human as not merely a physical entity, but a complex interwoven system of body, mind, heart, and energy.

Countries such as China, Japan, and a few European nations currently lead the way in the integration of modern and traditional practices. In modern Thailand, likewise, the state-of-the-art hospitals and the ancient traditions exist side by side in harmony. Most modern urban and rural Thais utilize the arts of massage, herbal healing, and spiritual healing in addition to modern medical technology from the West. The government of Thailand, in fact, is one of the biggest supporters of this blend of traditional and modern healing. In rural areas that remain far from Western hospitals, government-operated herbal clinics dispense tried-and-true traditional remedies alongside allopathic drugs with the support and blessing of the Thai government, the World Health Organization and UNICEF.

Herbal medicines are often thought to lack the effectiveness of over-the-counter and prescription allopathic medications and are sometimes considered to be mere placebos. In fact, natural substances form the basis of many of today's synthetic drugs, including aspirin, painkillers, and antibiotics. Many herbal medicines contain the same active ingredients as their allopathic counterparts and can be just as effective.

Herbal remedies may not have the immediate effect of Western drugs in treating acute disease or discomfort, but this is because they tend to work on the body as a whole rather than on any specific group of symptoms. Because the impact of any particular herb on the body is ameliorated by that herb's natural blend of complementary alkaloids, herbal medicines have a subtler effect on the system. One who is desensitized to these subtle effects due to years of use of pharmaceuticals, alcohol, nicotine, and caffeine may not initially notice the impact of herbs. However, through persistent use of herbal remedies, generally improving the diet, exercising, meditating, and living in harmony with the body and with nature, one will soon find that the cumulative benefits are not only noticeable, but indispensable!

Chapter II

The Theory of Royal Thai Herbalism

THE FOUR BODY ELEMENTS

The physical body, in the Thai system, is made up of the same four elements that permeate the entire universe: Earth, Water, Air, and Fire. The traditional Thai conception of these elements is roughly parallel to Ayurvedic cosmology. The Thais do not believe that there is literally a speck of earth, a drop of water, or a flame of fire in each atom of the universe; each element refers not to physical substance, but to the qualities of that substance. Substances that are solid can be said to have the qualities of the Earth element. Substances that are liquid are of the Water element. Movement is the quality of the Air element. Heat is the quality of the Fire element.

According to this conception, the organs of the human body can be broken down into categories.

THE FOUR BODY ELEMENTS, THEIR QUALITIES, AND THE ORGANS THEY AFFECT		
Element	Quality	Organs
Earth	Solid	Skin, muscle, tendon, bone, viscera, fat, other solid organs
Water	Liquid	Blood, eyes, phlegm, saliva, lymph, urine, semen, other liquids in the body
Air	Movement	Respiration, digestion, excretion, motion of the limbs and joints, sexuality, aging
Fire	Heat	Body temperature, circulatory system, metabolism

The constant interaction of the four elements gives rise to the processes of the human body and is the impetus behind physical life. It is of vital importance, therefore, to keep the four elements balanced throughout life. The elements can become unbalanced due to a variety of reasons. Environmental factors can affect the body, as for instance, when hot weather causes excess of the Fire element or rainy weather causes excess of the Water element. Food can also affect the balance, as for instance when indulgence in hot foods, sugar, and alcohol causes excess of the Fire element or indulgence in fatty and fried foods causes excess of the Earth element.

During the normal course of one's life, the elements go in and out of balance in a continuously changing state of health or disease. Children and the elderly are more susceptible to disease than average adults because of the delicate state of their elements. In children, the four elements are not yet fully mature, and in the elderly, they are weakened by many years of life. Gradually, the elements become more and more weak, and ultimately, when they are exhausted, the individual dies. The primary goal of traditional Thai dietary regimens and herbalism is to promote health and longevity by maintaining the vitality and balance of the four elements.

FOUR ELEMENT DIAGNOSTICS

According to Somchintana Ratarasarn,

> It is a must for an orthodox Thai doctor to have knowledge in the four elements... The basic principle of every branch of Thai medicine, particularly internal medicine, is the knowledge of the Four Body elements, their functions, and their interrelations which affect the health/sickness of the individual. The Four Body elements are regarded as the foundation of the whole body and the foundation of life.[5]

Diagnosing disease according to the four elements is thus a crucial part of Thai herbalism. Diagnostic skills take many years to develop, and traditionally, Thai apprentices studied under able teachers for decades before they were considered to be healers in their own right.

---

[5] Somchintana Ratarasarn, *The Principles and Concepts of Thai Classical Medicine* (Bangkok: Thai Khadi Research Institute, Thammasat University, 1986), 62.

Some basic guidelines can be outlined, however, using the chart on page 15:

- Imbalance of the Earth element would manifest as symptoms of the organs associated with the Earth element. Some examples would be: skin disease, bone disease, tumors, and other "solid" disorders.

- Imbalance of the Water element would manifest as symptoms of the organs associated with the Water element such as blood disease, eye disorders, renal disease, venereal disease, bladder or urinary tract infection or stones, and any diseases manifesting in abnormal urine or other liquid discharge. (It is interesting to note that diabetes is considered to be a Water element disease, and the two types of diabetes are known in Thai as "sweet-urine disease" and "bland-urine disease.")

- Imbalance of the Air element would manifest as symptoms of the organs associated with the Air element such as pneumonia, cough, mucous congestion, tuberculosis, bronchitis, other respiratory infections, fainting, dizziness, and arthritis. The Air element is considered to be the most important element in promoting mobility, strength, longevity, and vigor.

- Imbalance of the Fire element primarily manifests as diseases of the Fire element organs, the heart and circulatory system.

A complete picture of the organ system involved in the disease should be developed by asking questions, observing symptoms, and palpating the body of the patient. The Ayurvedic system of *tridosha* is frequently used to assist in diagnosis. (This is discussed in my book *The Spiritual Healing of Traditional Thailand*.) For those already familiar with the *Tridosha* system, this can be easily incorporated into Thai diagnosis by remembering that excessive *Vata* corresponds to excess of the Air element; excessive *Pitta* corresponds to excess of the Fire and Water elements; and excessive *Kapha* corresponds to excess of the Earth and Water elements.

Other common diagnostic techniques such as phrenology, reflexology, tongue diagnosis, and pulse diagnosis are also used by Thai healers, although they belong more properly to traditional Chinese medicine and represent later additions to the Thai system.

Once the affected organ system is pinpointed, the Thai healer would determine whether the disorder is manifesting as excess or depletion. Excess is typically accompanied by tightness, swelling, strong sharp pain, fever, skin eruptions, redness, fullness, high blood pressure, fast pulse, high body temperature, and radiation of symptoms in an outward direction. The excessive patient usually expresses anxiety, tension, irritability, shortness of temper and breath, and insomnia. Depletion, on the other hand, is typically accompanied by atrophy, emaciation, lack of appetite, dull aching pain, paleness, gauntness, emptiness, low blood pressure, slow pulse, low body temperature, and concentration of symptoms in an inward direction. The depleted patient usually feels weakness, dizziness, fatigue, sleepiness, and nausea.

Once the affected organ has been pinpointed, and it has been determined whether the disease is one of excess or depletion, the Thai herbalist will prescribe dietary changes and herbal supplements to either build or soothe this particular organ.

The newcomer to Thai herbalism should keep in mind the above points but should also recognize that even in allopathic medicine, diagnostic skill can sometimes be an art rather than a science. Symptoms can often appear as a mix of excess and depletion, and can appear in more than one organ system. For example, a patient with excessive Fire element may also exhibit depleted Air. This individual could manifest with heart disease, high blood pressure, high cholesterol, anxiety attacks, short temper, reddish color in the face, and a voracious appetite—all symptoms of Fire element excess. At the same time, he or she could exhibit chronic low-level lung infections, blocked sinuses, and a persistent cough—symptoms of Air depletion.

The Ten Tastes

Herbal medicines are traditionally broken down into ten "taste" classifications according to the primary taste of the herb. Since each element is associated with several organs and organ systems, and since each element is associated with several tastes, the tastes provide the link between diagnosis and herbal therapy. According to Trond and Schumacher,

> The taste rules are never elevated to being absolute and all-encompassing, but are regarded as "rules of thumb"... [nevertheless] the taste rules provide us in fact with the main links between theory and practice.[6]

The information in the chart opposite may be used to determine both the herbs and food which a patient should be given to help with an imbalance of elements and those which he or she should avoid to prevent further aggravation of such a condition.

---

6 Viggo Brun and Trond Schumacher, *Traditional Herbal Medicine in Northern Thailand* (Bangkok: White Lotus, 1994), 31.

THE TEN TASTES AND THEIR EFFECTS ON THE ELEMENTS		
Taste	Increases	Decreases
Astringent	Air	Earth, Water, Fire
Oily (Nutty)	Earth, Water, Fire	Air
Salty	Earth, Water, Fire	Air
Sweet	Earth, Water	Air, Fire
Bitter	Air	Earth, Water, Fire
Toxic (Nauseating)	Air, Fire	Earth, Water
Sour	Water, Fire	Earth, Air
Hot (Spicy)	Air, Fire	Earth, Water
Bland	Earth, Water, Air	Fire
Aromatic (Cool)	Earth, Water, Air	Fire

To continue with the example from the previous section, the excess Fire and depleted Air patient could be given astringent, sweet, bitter, bland and aromatic food and herbs to calm the Fire element, and would stay away from oily, salty, toxic, sour, and hot herbs and food in order not to build more Fire. Likewise, he or she could take astringent, bitter, toxic, hot, bland, and aromatic herbs and food to build the Air element, while staying away from oily, salty, sweet, and sour herbs and food to avoid depleting Air. When you put all of this together, considering the mixed symptoms the patient is exhibiting, it seems that the best course of action would be for the individual to take astringent, bitter, bland and aromatic herbs and food, and to avoid oily, salty, and sour herbs and food. Since the sweet, toxic, and hot tastes are indicated in one case and contraindicated in they other, they should probably be avoided as well. The chart on pages 20–22 illustrates some more connections between certain disorders and the ten tastes.

The tastes and some examples of food and herbs are listed in the chart *Herbs and Foods Classified by the Ten Tastes* on page 23. For more information on particular herbs and their uses, refer to the individual entries in the compendium of herbs (*Chapter VI* of this book).

In referring to the compendium and the indices, you will note that some herbs are listed in traditional sources in more than one taste category. This is most often due to the different tastes of different parts of the plant. For example, the lemon, kaffir lime, and common lime possess sour fruit and bitter rinds. Herbs may also be listed in multiple categories if they possess what Western herbalists call "double-action."

The Ten Tastes: Therapeutic Uses

This chart should be used as a general guideline. Individual entries in the herbal compendium should be consulted, as each herb has its own particular therapeutic uses.

Taste	Action	For Treatment of	Contraindications
Astringent	Hemostatic	Internal bleeding wounds	Constipation
	Topical astringent	Dysentery and other diarrhea	
	Topical antiseptic	Pus, discharge	
	Diuretic	Water retention	
	Hepatic	Liver and stomach disease	
	Digestive	Sluggish digestion	
	Stomachic		
	Antirheumatic	Arthritis	
Oily	Nutritive tonic	Impaired strength, energy, vitality	Obesity
		Chronically low body temperature	
		Stiff and sore joints, muscles, and tendons	
		Skin disease, itching	
Salty	Laxative	Constipation	Chronic thirst
	Antiseptic	Flatulence	Dehydration
		Sluggish digestion	
		Excessive mucous in digestive tract	
		Mouth sores	
Sweet	Nutritive tonic	Impaired strength energy, vitality	Diabetes
	Demulcent	Chronic disease, low immunity	Hypoglycemia
		Chronic fatigue exhaustion	Gum disease

Taste	Action	For Treatment of	Contraindications
Sweet, continued		Convalescence from disease or injury Asthma Sore throat, Cough	Tooth decay
Bitter	Bitter tonic Tonic for blood and bile Antipyretic Alterative Cholagogue Hepatic Lymphatic	Diseases of blood and bile Parasites and infection in blood Fever Dengue, malaria Low immune system	Chronic fatigue
Toxic	Detoxifier Anthelmintic Vermifuge Purgative Analgesic Antiseptic	Systemic infections Tetanus Venereal diseases Cholera, dysentery Diarrhea Gastro-intestinal parasites Infections Festering wounds	These herbs have a nauseating taste or smell, and should only be used with caution. Not prescribed for children or elderly patients.
Sour	Expectorant Pectoral Refrigerant Nervine Diuretic	Congested mucous Respiratory infections Asthma Bronchitis Cough Fever	

Taste	Action	For Treatment of	Contraindications
Sour, continued			
	General stimulant	Infection of blood, lymph	
		Sluggish circulation	
		Clarity of mind and senses	
Hot	General stimulant	Low immunity	Fever
	Digestive	Chronic fatigue	Hypertension
	Carminative	Sluggish digestion	Cardiac disease
	Cardiac	Indigestion	
	Expectorant	Flatulence	
	Aphrodisiac	Constipation	
	Anti-inflammatory	Sinusitis	
	Antispasmodic	Common cold, nasal congestion	
	Diaphoretic	Sore or cramping muscles	
Aromatic	Cardiac tonic	Heart disease	Aromatics are typically
	Hepatic	Circulatory problems	administered through
	Pectoral	Diseases of liver and lungs	sauna or steam, which
	Nervine	Chronic anxiety, tension, stress	should be avoided by
	Sedative	Hypertension	those suffering from
	Calmative	Psychological and emotional imbalances	fever, heart disease or
	Stimulant	Chronic fatigue, exhaustion	high blood pressure.
	Female tonic	Depression	Tea may be taken
		Mental clarity and well-being	instead.
		Post-partum depression	
Bland	Detoxifier	Food or chemical poisoning	
	Diuretic	Chronic thirst	

HERBS AND FOODS CLASSIFIED BY THE TEN TASTES

AROMATIC

Arabian Jasmine, *p.79*
Bulletwood, *p.84*
Camphor, *p.85*
Champaca, *p.90*
Damask Rose, *p.97*
Eucalyptus, *p.99*
Ironwood, *p.110*
Jasmine, *p.111*
Lemongrass, *p.113*
Lotus (flower), *p.116*
Night Jasmine, *p.122*
Peppermint, *p.127*
Sarapee, *p.133*
Ylang-Ylang, *p.144*

ASTRINGENT

Beleric Myrobalan,
   p.81
Catechu, *p.89*
Chebulic Myrobalan,
   p.91
Corkwood Tree, *p.96*
Golden Shower, *p.105*
Guava, *p.106*
Hanuman Prasan Kai,
   p.107
Hibiscus, *p.108*
Lacquer Tree, *p.113*
Mangosteen, *p.x118*
Oroxylum, *p.124*
Plantain, *p.128*
Pomegranate (fruit),
   p.129
Shorea, *p.135*
Turkish Rhubarb, *p.142*

BITTER

Alexandrian Senna,
   p.77
Aloe, *p.77*
Bitter Gourd, *p.82*

Boraphet, *p.107*
Candelabra Bush, *p.86*
Cassod Tree, *p.88*
Chiretta, *p.92*
Chrysanthemum, *p.92*
Cinchona, *p.93*
Crocodile Bile, *p.96*
False Daisy, *p.100*
Foetid Cassia, *p.100*
Gotu Kola, *p.105*
Green Tea, *p.106*
Henna, *p.107*
Ironweed, *p.110*
Kaffir Lime (rind),
   p.112
Lemon (rind), *p.113*
Lime (rind), *p.114*
Loog Thai Bai, *p.116*
Makaa, *p.117*
Mandarin Orange
   (rind), *p.117*
Mawaeng, *p.119*
Neem, *p.121*
Nutgrass, *p.123*
Sandalwood Tree,
   p.132
Soap Nut, *p.135*
Thai Caper, *p.139*
Tongkat Ali, *p.140*

BLAND

Alumina Clay, *p.78*
Banana, *p.81*
Caricature Plant, *p.87*
Ivy Gourd, *p.110*
Lime (root), *p.114*
Pumpkin, *p.130*
Purple Allamanda,
   p130
Ti Plant, *p.140*
Water Mimosa, *p.143*

HOT

Angelica, *p.78*
Asafoetida, *p.79*
Bael, *p.80*
Betel, *p.82*
Black Pepper, *p.83*
Calamus, *p.85*
Camphor, *p.85*
Cardamom, *p.87*
Cassumunar ginger,
   p.88
Cayenne, *p.90*
Chinese Chives, *p.91*
Cinnamon, *p.93*
Citronella Grass, *p.93*
Clove, *p.94*
Eucalyptus, *p.99*
Finger Root, *p.102*
Galangal, *p.103*
Garlic, *p.104*
Ginger, *p.105*
Ginseng, *p.106*
Holy Basil, *p.110*
Horseradish Tree, *p.111*
Lemongrass, *p.115*
Long Pepper, *p.117*
Musk, *p.122*
Nutmeg, *p.125*
Papaya (seed), *p.128*
Peppermint, *p.129*
Plumbago, *p.130*
Safflower, *p.134*
Star Anise, *p.138*
Turmeric, *p.143*
Wild Pepper Leaf, *p.145*
Zedoary, *p.146*
Zerumbet Ginger,
   p.146

OILY

Black Bean, *p.85*

Herbs and Foods Classified by the Ten Tastes, continued

Cashew Nut, *p.89*
Jackfruit (seed), *p.113*
Lotus (seed), *p.118*
Sesame Seeds, *p.136*
Tamarind (seed), *p.140*

SALTY

Baking Soda, *p.82*
Blue Crab, *p.85*
Cuttlefish, *p.98*
Ebony Tree (bark)
  p.100
Oyster, *p.127*
Sea Salt, *p.136*
Sting-Ray, *p.138*

SOUR

Alum Powder, *p.80*
Emblic Myrobalan,
  p.100
Gandaria, *p.103*
Kaffir Lime (fruit,
  leaf), *p.114*
Lemon (fruit), *p.115*

Lime (fruit), *p.116*
Mandarin Orange
  (juice), *p.119*
Mango, *p.120*
Otaheite Gooseberry,
  p.127
Pineapple, *p.129*
Pomelo, *p.131*
Somlom, *p.137*
Tamarind (fruit, leaf,
  bark), *p.140*

SWEET

Coconut, *p.97*
Ginseng, *p.106*
Honey, *p.111*
Licorice, *p.116*
Longan, *p.117*
Milk, Raw, *p.121*
Pandanus, *p.127*
Papaya (fruit), *p.128*
Star Anise, *p.138*
Stevia, *p.138*

Sugar Apple (fruit)
  p.139
Sugar Cane, *p.139*
Sugar Palm, *p.140*
Woolly Grass, *p.145*

TOXIC

Combretum, *p.97*
Datura, *p.99*
Ebony (fruit, root),
  p.100
Marijuana, *p.120*
Monkey Jack, *p.121*
Opium Poppy, *p.126*
Pomegranate (root)
  p.131
Rangoon Creeper,
  p.133
Sugar Apple (leaf and
  seed), *p.139*
Sulfur, *p.140*
Thong Phan Chang,
  p.141
Toothbrush Tree, *p.143*

Herbs with double-action have the ability to both stimulate and relax. They act to regulate the body and mind by balancing excessive or depleted energy. Thai herbs that possess the qualities of double-action include Camphor, Eucalyptus, Ginseng, Lemongrass, Peppermint, and Star Anise.

CLASSIFICATION OF HERBS BY ACTION

Many readers will be familiar with the classification by action used in Western herbalism. In addition to the ten tastes, a second classification system exists within traditional Thai herbalism which closely parallels the Western method. This system classifies herbs strictly by their action on the body, not by any property of the herb itself. Used in conjunction with the tastes, the classification by action can give the herbalist a full picture of the therapeutic benefits of a particular herb.

The Thai system of classification by action includes the following major categories.[7] For a complete list of herbs by their action, see the *Index by Action* at the end of this book.

Anthelmintic and **vermifuge** herbs destroy and expel tapeworms, bacteria, yeast, and other parasites from the digestive tract. They usually possess laxative qualities as well but are sometimes taken in combination with more powerful purgatives to effectively expel the parasites.

Anti-inflammatory herbs are used topically to lessen inflammation caused by bruises, contusions, sprains, and other internal injuries, as well as inflammation associated with boils, animal bites, and contact with poisonous plants or insects such as bees and scorpions.

Antipyretic herbs are used primarily to bring down fevers and accompanying symptoms like chronic thirst and fever blisters. These herbs are mainly used to control symptoms and are generally combined with purgatives to expel disease. Bitter antipyretics are known in Western herbalism as bitter tonics. (See also Tonics.)

Aphrodisiac herbs heighten sexual potency and arousal in either sex. These herbs function by stimulating and strengthening bodily functions and therefore may also serve as stimulants and tonics. Most stimulants and tonics are also, conversely, aphrodisiacs. (See also Male and Female Tonics.)

Astringent herbs (not to be confused with the classification of astringent taste discussed in the previous section, although there is much overlap) have the effect of drying up bodily secretions and discharges. They are used internally to counter diarrhea, dysentery, and internal bleeding, or externally to cleanse the skin and promote healing of wounds. They should not be used in the case of food or chemical poisoning, when the body's natural impulse is to purge these toxins.

---

[7] For ease of readability, I have not used the Thai language in classifying these herbs. Instead, I have relied upon the work of Somchintana Ratarasarn, who has translated these categories into English and has shown how many of these categories are roughly interchangeable with their Western counterparts. Much of the information in this section is from his book, *The Principles and Concepts of Thai Classical Medicine*. It should be noted that some of the herbs in this collection have not been fully evaluated by Western herbalists, and therefore may never have been classified before anywhere else. When faced with this situation, I have taken the Thai tradition at its word and classified the plant accordingly. That is to say, for example, that if Thai traditional medicine uses a particular plant as an anthelmintic, in this book I have classified it as such.

Carminative and **antacid** herbs are used to dispel gas from the digestive tract. Carminatives work on the lower intestines, for cases of flatulence and bloated bowels. For cases of heartburn, gastritis, and other ailments of the upper digestive tract, see Stomachics.

Cholagogue herbs treat diseases of the gall bladder. They stimulate the production of bile and are thus useful for treatment of chronic intestinal problems. Traditionally, disorder of the bile is held to be the physical cause of psychological symptoms such as delirium and hallucination.

Diuretic herbs are used traditionally to treat any disease in which the urine becomes abnormal. These herbs help dispel toxins from the body by promoting urination and have a tonifying and strengthening effect on the kidneys. Diuretics are used in treatment of kidney stones and other disorders of the kidneys and bladder, for obesity, water-retention, and gout (caused by build-up of uric acid). They are also used for diabetes. Diuretics should not be used in patients that exhibit constipation.

Emetic herbs cause vomiting. Many herbs are emetic at toxic levels, but some are non-toxic emetics, which can be useful for purging the stomach. Emetics are also used to purge severe congestion or infection of the chest, bronchi, and sinuses by the catharsis of vomiting.

Emmenagogues regulate the menstrual cycle. They are used for all gynecological problems in which the first sign is the abnormality of the menses (abnormal color, timing, duration, amount, etc.), which Thai medicine considers to be an indication of the general state of health of the reproductive system as a whole. Many of these herbs can also be used for uterine infections, cysts, tumors, and cancers as they increase the flow of blood and promote regular function of the female reproductive system. Emmenagogues are also used to enhance fertility.

Expectorant herbs encourage the expulsion of mucous from the body. They are particularly useful in treatment of colds with congestion, sinus congestion, and mucous build-up in the stomach and bowels. Most expectorants are also antitussives, used to treat coughs.

Hepatics are herbs that have a beneficial effect on the liver. These are used in treatment of disorders and malfunctions of the liver caused by internal injury, toxicity, cirrhosis, and hepatitis.

Pectoral herbs tonify and strengthen the respiratory organs.

Purgatives and **alteratives** are herbs which cleanse the organs, purify the blood, and detoxify the tissues, bringing health and vitality to the body. Some purgatives are mild laxatives that can be used occasionally in fasting and for general constipation. Some have stronger laxative qualities and are used for vigorous cleansing of the bowels. Alteratives have no laxative quality but have a detoxifying effect on the stomach, kidneys, bladder, and blood. Purgatives and alteratives are used in treatment of systemic infection, parasites, or disease, for fevers, contagious viral and bacterial diseases, cancers, and in cases of food or chemical poisoning. They should not be used by pregnant women, children, the elderly, or extremely weak or chronically exhausted patients, as they may lack the strength required for detoxification.

Refrigerants are herbs which lower the body's temperature. They are used traditionally to lower fevers, and usually make great cold drinks in the summertime.

Sedatives and **calmatives** are used to counteract psycho-physiological disturbances such as stress, insomnia, heart palpitations, panic attacks, and severe anxiety. These herbs range in effect from mild (jasmine) to pronounced (opium) and are prescribed according to severity of symptoms.

Stimulants heighten all of the physiological processes of the body. They encourage digestion, enhance the senses, and tonify the immune system. Stimulants are often used as adjuvants (helping herbs), especially in diseases where weakness or fatigue is prevalent.

• **Cardiac Stimulants** are tonics for the heart. They are used to counter hypotension and to increase strength and vitality of the heart muscle, circulation, and veins. Stimulants should be avoided by those with high blood pressure or chronic anxiety.

Stomachics encourage the proper function of the upper digestive system. Stomachics are used to treat indigestion, peptic ulcer, gastritis, and other disorders of the stomach. These herbs increase the appetite and are used often in cases of cachexia (the general emaciation, weakness, and physical wasting associated with long-term chronic diseases). By stimulating digestion they allow the body to better assimilate nutrients, and are therefore useful for many types of disease, as well as for promoting general health and vigor.

Tonics are herbs that strengthen the body, encourage immunity, and promote the natural healing process.

- **Nutritive Tonics** are used to treat emaciation, weakness, fatigue, and paralysis, and are especially prescribed during convalescence from chronic or long-term illness. Many of these tonics have specific effects on the immune, the nervous, and the reproductive systems. Nutritive tonics are useful as adjuvants (helping herbs) in any treatment for chronic disease and are also useful as daily supplements for children and the elderly.

- **Female Tonics** are herbs which strengthen the female reproductive organs. Some are prescribed to enhance fertility or to regulate the menstrual cycle; some are especially given to strengthen uterine function during pregnancy, while others are used to tonify and heal the reproductive system immediately after giving birth.

- **Male Tonics** are used to treat male impotence, premature ejaculation, and other male sexual dysfunction.

- **Blood Tonics** and **Lymphatics** are used to treat what in Thai is called "bad blood" and "bad lymph". These are generalized states of infection or toxicity that manifest in symptoms such as rashes, acne, boils, and other skin eruptions, pale skin, fainting spells, fatigue, and frequent or recurring fevers. Malaria and other blood-borne parasites would fall under this category, as would blood poisoning, leukemia, and lymphatic cancer. Animal blood is sometimes called for in remedies, especially that of the rhinoceros, horse, and the langur monkey, but there are many herbal medicines as well.

Vulnerary and **Emmolient** herbs are used topically to promote the healing of wounds and burns of the skin. These herbs may be used externally as topical salves and balms, or internally for treatment of internal injuries, bruising, and hemorrhage.

WESTERN CLASSIFICATION OF HERBS

In compiling this collection, I have found it useful to include several classifications that are not properly part of the traditional Thai system. These are terms common to Western herbalism, and while there may be some degree of overlap with the preceding classes, they are used in this collection side by side with traditional Thai terminology for ease of reference.

I have taken the liberty of classifying many of the herbs in this collection in accordance with these Western categories in addition to the traditional Thai categories. For example, if Thai medicine prescribes an herb to combat nausea, I have listed it as an antiemetic—even though this category does not exist in traditional Thai classification—in order to assist the Western herbalist using this book as a reference. (For a complete list of herbs by their action, see *Index by Action*.)

Analgesic herbs lessen pain. Most can be used both internally and topically. The pain-relieving properties of the plants listed in this collection range from anodynes such as cloves to potent anesthetics like opium. Analgesics should always be administered internally with care, as they may have a pronounced physiological effect.

Antiallergic herbs are natural antihistamines which soothe the symptoms of hayfever-like allergies.

Antiemetic herbs treat symptoms of nausea and vomiting.

Antioxidants are herbs containing high levels of oxidation-retarding compounds such as vitamins A and C. These herbs are naturally detoxifying and contribute to long-term health, immunity, and longevity.

Antipruritics calm itchiness of the skin associated with allergic reactions and rashes.

Antirheumatic herbs are used to soothe joint pain and inflammation and are especially used for cases of arthritis, chronic back pain, and repetitive stress injuries.

Antiseptics are used on the surface of the skin to treat ulcers, sores, bacterial infections, fungus, parasites, and other skin diseases. Many of the herbs listed under this category may be used orally as well for tooth and gum disease, cold sores, and abscesses.

Antispasmodic herbs counteract spasms and muscular cramps. Many are used in conjunction with expectorants and/or antitussives to treat severe cases of cough, and some act as bronchodilators useful in treating asthmatics.

Antitumor herbs have been shown to shrink or halt the growth of cysts and tumors. Many of these traditional herbs are being researched for beneficial effects against cancers of all types.

Antitussives are herbs which soothe cough, sore throat, and other cold symptoms.

Appetizers improve appetite. They are useful to overcome wasting diseases, emaciation, and lack of hunger. Many are also digestives, which promote the digestive function.

Bitter Tonics stimulate the digestion, the immune system, the blood, and the internal organs. They have particularly beneficial effects on the liver and bile. They provide general detoxification, blood cleansing, internal antibacterial action, and aid in convalescence from persistent or chronic diseases. They are also important in the treatment of cancer, tumors, hepatitis, diabetes, blood diseases, and systemic infections.

Bronchodilators open the bronchi and other respiratory passages. These are used to treat disorders, inflammations, and infections of the respiratory system, colds with chest congestion, bronchitis, tuberculosis, and especially, asthma.

Demulcent herbs soothe irritations of membranes with a moistening effect. They can be used internally in cases of dry cough or externally for irritations, dry or chapped skin, burns, and dry hair.

Diaphoretic herbs promote sweating, usually by raising the body temperature. They are useful to break a fever, to warm the body, and to dispel toxins through the pores. Due to their detoxifying action, diaphoretics are used to treat colds, flu, skin diseases, rheumatism, and lymph problems.

Digestives promote digestion and assimilation of foods by encouraging the body's natural digestive processes and by aiding in the breaking down of foods in the gastrointestinal tract.

Galactogogue herbs increase the production and/or quality of breast milk.

Hemostatic herbs are used internally or externally to halt bleeding.

Laxative herbs are intestinal stimulants. They have a milder effect than purgatives on the bowels and are useful for symptomatic treatment of constipation.

Chapter III

Every-day Herbs

FOOD THERAPY, OR EVERY-DAY MEDICINE

Medicinal herbs found throughout this collection are ingested every day in the typical Thai diet. In fact, the Thai herbalist traditionally will recommend modifications to the diet before recommending more powerful herbal medicines. Every herb—and in fact everything we eat—has an effect on our bodies and minds. In traditional Thai cuisine, almost every dish is considered to be therapeutic. An old Thai proverb says that all diseases originate in the food we eat. In the West, we also say "You are what you eat." If we eat well, we will enjoy health, well-being, and longevity; if we eat poorly, we will become unhealthy, unhappy, and prone to illness.

According to legend, when the Father Doctor Jivaka was a young man, he was given his final examination by his master. He was challenged to go off into the forest and find a plant that could not be used as a medicine. After searching the world, Jivaka returned and declared to his teacher, "Everything is medicine!" At that point the old master knew that his student had completed his training.

It is with this philosophy that traditional healers have approached the world over thousands of years, and it is this philosophy that continues to form the backbone of the traditional Thai medical system.

THE ENERGETICS OF FOOD

Every food, drink, and condiment—whether it be plant, animal, or mineral—can be classified by a predominance of one of the ten tastes, and therefore can be used as medicine. Referring back to the charts in *Chapter II*, you can determine which foods are most likely to assist in treatment of specific disorders and which should be avoided.

Below are some foods listed by taste:

Taste	Example Foods
Astringent	Guava (unripe), Pomegranate, Rhubarb
Oily (Nutty)	Beans, Butter, Nuts, Oils, Seeds
Salty	Seafood, Sea Salt
Sweet	Coconut, Dairy, Fruit, Honey, Sugars
Bitter	Chrysanthemum, Green Tea, Leafy Greens
Sour	Citrus Fruits and Juices
Hot (Spicy)	Anise, Basil, Cayenne, Cinnamon, Cloves, Garlic, Ginger, Lemongrass, most Meats, Nutmeg, Peppermint, Turmeric
Bland	Banana, Gourds, Pumpkin, Squashes, Bland White Vegetables (e.g. Daikon, Potato)
Aromatic (Cool)	Edible Flowers, Jasmine Tea, Lotus Root

GLOBAL RECOMMENDATIONS

In modern times, Jivaka's motto that everything is medicine should be slightly re-interpreted. Certain man-made foods commonly available are so toxic to the system that I would argue they don't have enough redeeming nutritional or medicinal qualities to offset the dangers. Herbalists, natural healers, and nutritionists the world over agree that the following modern foods and additives should be on everyone's list of items to avoid:

Refined white sugar: This is a poison to the liver and kidneys; it overtaxes the metabolic system and its use can lead to diabetes and eventual organ failure. Use honey, raw sugar, or stevia as a substitute.

Bleached white flour: This overprocessed food is extremely common in the West. Bleached flour not only contains high levels of potentially toxic chemicals used in processing, but has been stripped of almost all of its nutritional value (which then is added back in to make "enriched flour"). White flour breaks down into sugar in the digestive system, and leads to the same conditions. Furthermore, white flour is exceedingly difficult for the digestive tract to handle, leading to sluggish digestion and depletion of the Air and Fire elements. Use unbleached white or whole wheat flour instead.

Milk: Unless it is raw, milk is another case of an overprocessed food. What nutritional value milk has is rendered unusable by the homogenization process, and is typically added back in after processing. The vitamin D touted by the dairy industry is usually an additive and can just as easily be taken in a multivitamin or through other foods. The dairy industry is also a leading user of hormones and antibiotics, which can enter the human system and potentially cause long-term damage to the endocrine and immune systems. Use raw milk or yogurt instead, organic dairy products, or dairy substitutes such as soy, almond, or rice milk.

Hydrogenated Oil: With a chemical composition close to plastic, hydrogenated oils are some of the most dangerous and potentially carcinogenic substances in our foods. Hydrogenation is usually for consistency or texture, as food companies believe it makes the food appear less greasy than whole oil. The process renders beneficial oils useless to the body, and hydrogenated oils are immediately stored as fat. Look for alternative hydrogenation-free products at your local health food store.

Artificial Colors, Flavors, and Preservatives: If you read the labels on your food purchases, you will realize that the typical Western adult consumes chemical food additives in every meal. These unnatural ingredients are both unhealthy and unnecessary. Look for alternative 100% natural foods at your local health food store.

When looking at the typical American diet, you may notice that many of us eat items from this list in every meal. In fact, some "American classics"—such as hamburger, fries, and a Coke from a fast-food chain or Froot Loops and milk or peanut butter and jelly on white bread for breakfast—are almost totally made up of these items.

Everyone should try to limit junk food intake, especially the very young and the very old, who lack the strength to deal with these toxins. Overeating these foods can result in serious disorders. According to the Thai theories of the elements and tastes, most junk foods are sweet foods, which deplete the Air element, leading to depletion of digestion, sexuality, and motion, and increasing the effects of aging. Hydrogenated oils, as oily foods, additionally cause aggravation of the Fire element, leading to heart and circulatory disease. Because of their refined processing, these foods affect the body much more strongly than natural sweet and oily foods, which can be used medicinally.

DIETARY REGIMENS FOR HEALTH AND LONGEVITY

The following are recommendations from the Wat Po texts regarding specific dietary regimens for different age groups. These suggestions are accompanied by a list of foods from this compendium which are easily found in most Western supermarkets, Asian food stores, or herbal supply shops.

- Children to age 16 should consume more sweet and sour herbs to ward off childhood illnesses, colds, and coughs.

  Recommended herbal supplements for children's diet: Anise, Honey, Gooseberry, Lemon, Licorice, Lime, Longan, Raw Milk, Pineapple, Tamarind

- Adults aged 16–32 should consume more astringent, salty, bitter and sour herbs for vitality, healthy blood and bile.

  Recommended herbal supplements for adult diet: Aloe Juice, Bitter Gourd, Chiretta, Chrysanthemum, Gooseberry, Green Tea, Lemon, Lime, Orange Rind, Pineapple, Pomegranate, Seafood, Tamarind

- Adults 32 years and over should consume more hot, bitter, salty, astringent, and aromatic herbs.

  Recommended herbal supplements for middle-age adult diet: Aloe Juice, Basil, Bitter Gourd, Black Pepper, Cardamom, Cayenne, Chiretta, Chrysanthemum, Cinnamon, Clove, Garlic, Ginger, Green Tea, Jasmine, Lemongrass, Lotus, Orange Rind, Pomegranate, Seafood, Turmeric, all Bitter Tonics

- Special herbs are recommended as part of the diet of older adults (50 and up) for strength, longevity, and the heart.

  Recommended herbal supplements for older adult diet (in addition to middle-age adult suggestions): Asafoetida, Gingko, Ginseng, Gotu Kola, Honey, Jackfruit, Reishi, Papaya, Safflower, Sesame

DIETARY REGIMENS FOR THE SEASONS

Traditional Thai herbalists also advocate diet modifications depending on the season. The following are some recommendations from the Wat Po texts:

- In the hot season, individuals should consume more bitter foods, which are cooling to the system and relieve Fire element diseases.

  Recommended hot season foods: Aloe Juice, Bitter Gourd, Chiretta, Chrysanthemum, Green Tea, Orange Rind

- In the rainy season, one should ingest more foods of the hot taste, which alleviate the effects of Water.

  Recommended rainy season foods: Basil, Black Pepper, Cardamom, Cayenne, Cinnamon, Clove, Garlic, Ginger, Lemongrass, Turmeric

- In the cold season, sour foods are recommended to stimulate the Fire element.

  Recommended cold season foods: Gooseberry, Lemon, Lime, Pineapple, Tamarind

Since most of the West has four, rather than three, seasons, some re-interpretation is necessary if we are to apply these principles to our own yearly cycles. The hot season and cold season clearly correspond to our summer and winter, and many areas of the U.S. and Europe have what could be considered a rainy season in the springtime. However, some flexibility will be required when using these recommendations outside of Southeast Asia.

In addition to food recommendations for the three Thai seasons, there are traditional herbal remedies associated with each as well. These are described in detail in the list of medicinal recipes in *Chapter V*.

Dietary Regimens for Specific Disorders

The chart on the next page gives recommended daily food therapy for specific diseases, disorders, and physical ailments from the Wat Po texts (additional suggestions can be found by referring to the *Index by Application* at the end of this book).

Thai Recipes for Health and Harmony

Rich in spices and covering a wide gamut of flavors, Thai cuisine is noted for its often surprising combination of tastes. A Thai curry will be pungent, spicy, and sweet. A dessert may be sweet and salty at the same time, with an aromatic twist. These interesting and unusual combination of flavors have made Thai food one of the most popular Asian cuisines in the world.

There are several reasons as to why tropical cultures around the globe usually develop more herb-laden cuisines than their temperate counterparts. One reason is certainly food preservation. All pre-modern societies used techniques such as smoking, pickling, fermenting, and drying to preserve food, but in hot climates where food spoils quickly, these methods of preservation were elevated almost to an art form. Throughout the equatorial regions of the world, where spices are more plentiful, one still finds the frequent use of such

DAILY FOOD THERAPY FOR SPECIFIC DISEASES AND DISORDERS	
Condition	Food Recommendations
Allergies	Pumpkin, Squashes, Bland White Vegetables (e.g. Daikon, Potato)
Blood Disorders and Diseases	Aloe Juice, Bitter Gourd, Garlic, Kaffir Lime, Longan, Mango, Pineapple, Turmeric
Chronic Constipation, Sluggish Digestion	Basil, Black Pepper, Cayenne, Cloves, Galangal, Ginger, Lemongrass, Papaya, Seafood, Tamarind
Heart Disease, Hypertension	Jasmine, Lotus
Kidney Disorders	Ginger, Green Tea, Kaffir Lime, Papaya, Pineapple
Rheumatism, Weak Joints, Underdeveloped Muscles	Black Bean, Butter, Cashew Nut, Lotus Seed, Oils, Sesame Seed, Tamarind
Weakness, Fatigue	Cashew Nut, Cayenne, Dairy, Garlic, Honey, Jackfruit, Longan, Lotus, Meat, Melon, Sugar Cane

herbs as garlic, ginger, and chili to aid in food preservation. In Southeast Asia, a wide range of this type of food is still consumed in the villages, where electrification is recent and refrigeration is rare. The rural Thai diet includes such favorites as mangoes pickled in chili paste, dried bananas preserved in honey, fermented fish paste, and other strong-tasting delicacies that are bizarre (and sometimes distasteful) to the Western palate.

Another reason for heavy use of spices is the medicinal qualities of these spices themselves. Not only do many herbs prevent bacteria from spoiling the food, but they are a type of daily "food therapy" to ward off illness. In the tropics, where the climate is more conducive to bacterial, fungal, and viral infections, it seems only natural that the cuisine would include larger quantities of antibacterial herbs and spices. To give an example, *tom yam*, a popular Thai soup, is an excellent remedy for flu, intestinal trouble, and the common cold—sort of the Thai equivalent of Mom's chicken soup. In looking at the main ingredients (galangal, kaffir lime leaves, garlic, chili) one finds that all of these herbs are effective decongestants, antitussives, and antibacterials.

The following are recipes for Thai dishes that particularly embody the principles of "food therapy." Most of these recipes are traditional favorites from the Chiang Mai Thai Cookery School (see *Bibliography* for more information).

Main Dishes

TOM YAM

One of the most popular dishes in Thailand, *tom yam* soup is the quintessential therapeutic dish, calling for a blend of spices that consists of many herbs recognized around the world as powerful tonics and antibiotics. This is a very soothing meal for colds, flu, and intestinal trouble.

> *300 g prawns, washed, peeled, and de-veined (for vegetarian*
> *version, use silken tofu)*
> *750 ml chicken or vegetable stock*
> *6 cloves garlic, crushed*
> *6 shallots, sliced*
> *2 stalks lemongrass, white portion only, sliced into one inch pieces*
> *10 thin slices of galangal, skin removed*
> *200 g straw mushrooms, cut in half*
> *8 cherry tomatoes, halved*
> *20 small green chilies, halved lengthwise (use less for mild*
> *spice)*
> *3 tbs (45 ml) fish sauce or soy sauce*
> *5 kaffir lime leaves, de-stemmed*
> *2 tbs (30 ml) lime juice*
> *10 g cilantro, chopped*

Put stock, garlic, shallots, lemongrass, and galangal in large stockpot and bring to a boil. Add mushrooms and tomatoes, and bring back to a boil. Add chilies, fish sauce, and kaffir lime leaves. Cook over medium heat for 2 minutes. Add prawns and cook for 1 more minute. Remove from heat, and add lime juice. Garnish with cilantro before serving. (Serves 4)

Note: In this soup, pieces of lemongrass, galangal, and chilies, are served but not eaten.

PAD THAI

Thailand's national dish. Whether it is served in a five-star hotel or in a banana-leaf plate from a street vendor, this noodle dish is a favorite among Thais and tourists alike.

> *300 g rice noodles, pre-soaked in lukewarm water for at least*
> *30 minutes*
> *2 eggs, beaten*

120 g tofu, chopped small and pre-fried until crisp
20 g chives, chopped in 1-inch pieces
60 g bean sprouts
3 tbs (45 ml) peanut oil
1 tbs chopped garlic
1 tbs dried shrimp (optional)
3 tbs palm sugar or raw sugar (optional)
3 tbs (45 ml) fish sauce or soy sauce
3 tbs peanuts, chopped
1 lime, cut into wedges
3 tbs cilantro

Fry garlic and shrimp in oil until brown. Add rice noodles, stirring over high heat 3 minutes until noodles are soft. Add eggs, sugar, fish or soy sauce, sprouts, chives, tofu, and peanuts, stirring briskly to combine. Remove from heat as soon as eggs are well cooked. Serve garnished with lime wedges and cilantro. (Serves 2 as main dish, or 4–5 as appetizer.)

Gaen Kaew Wan

A spicy, rich green curry that is 100% Thai. To simplify this recipe, buy green curry paste from any grocery that sells Thai food.

300 g chicken breast (use extra-firm tofu or tempeh as
vegetarian substitute)
3–4 tbs green curry paste (use only 2–3 tbs if store-bought)
250 ml coconut cream
250 ml coconut milk
3 Chinese eggplants (the long thin variety), cut into 1/2 inch
pieces
40 g palm sugar (optional)
2 tbs (30 ml) fish sauce
2 kaffir lime leaves, de-stemmed
30 g sweet basil
1 green chili, sliced
1 red chili, sliced

Curry Paste Ingredients:
1 tsp coriander seeds, dry-roasted
1/2 tsp cumin seeds, dry-roasted
1/2 tsp black peppercorns
1/2 tsp salt (Note that when I use vegetarian paste, I have had to
add more salt to the recipe, due to the lack of salty shrimp
paste.)
1 tsp galangal, chopped and skin removed
3 tbs lemongrass, white part only, chopped
1 tsp kaffir lime leaf, chopped

2 tbs coriander root
2 tbs shallots, chopped
1 tbs garlic
1 tsp shrimp paste (or vegetarian substitute)
1 tsp turmeric, chopped and skin removed
20 small green chilies
30 g sweet basil leaves

To make curry paste, grind dried ingredients with mortar and pestle or in coffee grinder. Mash all other ingredients with mortar and pestle, or in food processor. Mixed dry with wet ingredients, and set aside.

Put 220 ml coconut cream into a wok and fry for 3–5 minutes, stirring continuously. Add green curry paste and fry for 1–2 minutes. Add chicken, and cook until white. Add palm sugar, fish sauce, thin coconut milk, and eggplant; bring to boil. Cook 4–5 minutes until eggplant is slightly soft. Add kaffir lime leaves and half of the basil leaves. Remove from heat. Garnish with chilies, remaining basil, and remaining coconut cream. (Serves 4)

NAM PRIK GAENG PED

Green curry's sister dish, the famous Thai red curry. Again, to simplify preparation, buy red curry paste from any store that sells Asian foods.

250 g fish, boned and cut into bite-sized pieces (use butternut
*   squash as vegetarian substitute)*
3 tbs (45 ml) sesame or peanut oil
4 tbs red curry paste (use only 2 tbs if store-bought)
750 ml coconut milk
2 large eggplants, cut into bite-sized pieces
100 g bamboo shoots, cut into bite-sized pieces
2 tbs (30 ml) fish or soy sauce
3 kaffir lime leaves, de-stemmed
2 large red chilies, seeds removed and sliced
basil leaves

Curry Paste Ingredients:
1 tsp galangal, skinned and grated
2 tsp lemongrass, white part only
1 tsp kaffir lime peel (leaves may be substituted)
1 tsp coriander root
1 tbs coriander seeds, roasted till brown
2 cardamom pods, roasted till brown
1 tsp salt (Note that when I use vegetarian paste, I have had
*   to add more salt to the recipe, due to the lack of salty*
*   shrimp paste.)*
1 tsp black peppercorns
3 tbs chopped shallots

3 tbs chopped garlic
1 tsp shrimp paste
10 large dried red chilies, seeds removed and soaked in water
  for 10 minutes
10 small red Thai chilies (also sometimes called bird's eye
  chilies.)

To make curry paste, powder dried ingredients with mortar and pestle or in coffee grinder. Mash all other ingredients with mortar and pestle, or in food processor. Mixed dry with wet ingredients, and set aside.

Fry curry paste in oil over high heat for 3 minutes. Add coconut milk and boil. Add eggplant and bamboo shoots; simmer for 4 minutes. Add fish sauce, kaffir lime leaves, and fish. Cook for 2 minutes until fish is done. Serve garnished with large chilies and basil leaves. (Serves 4)

BITTER GOURD STIR-FRY

A tonic widely recommended by Thai herbalists, the bitter gourd is accompanied in this dish by hot herbs that encourage digestion and detoxification. (For vegetarian version, substitute soy for fish and oyster sauce.)

200 g bitter gourd, chopped in $^1/_2$ inch pieces (chopped
  zucchini, squash, pumpkin, mushrooms, or green beans
  may be substituted)
100 g extra-firm tofu (crumbled tempeh, scrambled eggs, or
  ground pork may be substituted)
4 tbs (60 ml) sesame oil
6 cloves garlic, chopped
1 small onion, diced
60 g shredded ginger
60 g spring onions
2 tbs (30 ml) light soy sauce
2 tbs (30 ml) fish sauce
3 tbs (45 ml) oyster sauce
2 red chilies, sliced
120 ml chicken stock or water
4 tbs chopped basil

Prepare tofu by boiling in water for 10–15 minutes until firm. Let cool, and crumble by hand. If using tempeh, eggs, or pork, brown in sauteé pan with a small amount of sesame oil.

Heat oil in wok or sauté pan. Fry garlic until brown. Add onion and ginger; cook until soft. Add bitter gourd, tofu, sauces, chili, and water or chicken stock; cook 2–3 minutes. Garnish with basil before serving. (Serves 4)

SOM TAM

Som tam, also known as "pok-pok" for the sound of the mortar and pestle when making it, is the most popular street-vendor meal in northern Thailand, and is wonderful for stimulation of the digestion. The recipe calls for unripe papaya, which is a rich source of digestive enzymes, but this dish is delicious when substituting unripe mango, raw zucchini, carrots, summer squash, cabbage, or cucumber. When ordering this dish in Thailand, it may come garnished with fermented soft-shelled crab.

> *200 g unripe papaya, peeled and grated into thin strips*
> *3 cloves garlic*
> *10 small green chilies*
> *1/4 cup (approx 60 g) green beans, cut in 1 inch pieces*
> *2 tbs dried shrimp*
> *2 tbs (30 ml) fish sauce or soy sauce*
> *2 tbs (30 ml) lime juice*
> *1 tsp palm sugar*
> *4 cherry tomatoes, halved*
> *2 tbs peanuts, roasted*

Put garlic, chilies, and beans into mortar and pound with pestle. Add papaya and bruise. Add dried shrimp, fish sauce, lime juice, and palm sugar, and stir well. Stir in tomatoes and peanuts. Serve cold with sticky rice on bed of lettuce or cabbage. (Serves 2)

MIXED MUSHROOMS

A popular dish in Northern Thailand during the rainy season, when a wide variety of wild mushrooms pop up in the mountains. Sesame oil is the key to a light and healthy stir-fry. Serve over rice, or mix into plain noodles to make Asian pasta primavera. (For vegetarian version, substitute soy for fish and oyster sauce.)

> *3 tbs (45 ml) sesame oil*
> *3 cloves garlic, chopped*
> *1 onion, sliced*
> *100 g mixed wild mushrooms*
> *100 g straw mushrooms, halved*
> *6 baby-corn, cut in half, and split lengthwise*
> *125 ml chicken stock or water*
> *1 red chili, sliced lengthwise into thin strips*
> *4 spring onions, sliced into 1 inch pieces*
> *1 tbs (15 ml) fish sauce*
> *1 tbs (15 ml) soy sauce*
> *1 tbs (15 ml) oyster sauce*

1 tsp tapioca flour dissolved in 3 tbs water
¹/2 cup (approx. 20 g) cilantro, chopped

Heat oil in wok; fry garlic over high heat until brown. Add onion and stir fry till clear. Add mushrooms and stir-fry 1 minute. Add baby-corn and stock; cook till soft. Add chili, spring onions, and sauces; simmer until vegetables are cooked. Remove from heat. Immediately stir in tapioca flour, and allow sauce to thicken. Serve garnished with cilantro. (Serves 2)

Appetizers

THAI PAAN

An Indian favorite, paans are betel nut preparations with a stimulating effect not unlike caffeine. Indian paans typically include dozens of bizarre ingredients such as gold leaf, quicklime, and even opium. The edible Thai version of the paan is much more tame (and tasty!). A favorite appetizer in Thailand, this paan is a cornucopia of medicinal herbs, a fun hors d'oeuvre, and an instant "taste of Thailand."

Use any or all of the following:
betel leaf (lettuce may be used as a substitute)
peanuts, roasted and salted
coconut, shredded and toasted
lime rind, chopped into ¹/8 inch segments
ginger, shredded
garlic, minced
fresh cayenne peppers, minced (remove seeds for milder spice)
raisins
starfruit, diced
cashews, roasted and salted

Dipping sauce ingredients:
1 part honey
1 part water
cilantro, chopped
dried cracked red chili to taste

Typically, this dish is served by placing small bowls with each individual ingredient around a central plate of betel or lettuce leaves. Paan is made by wrapping lettuce around any or all of the other ingredients. Serve paans with a dipping sauce or the sweet chili sauce shown on page 43.

CHICKEN IN PANDANUS LEAVES

The pandanus palm is used in herbal medicine as a heart tonic, an antipyretic, and a diuretic. In this dish, the leaves are not eaten but are used in the cooking process.

> *200 g chicken breast, tofu, or tempeh, cut into 20 two-inch pieces*
> *20 pandanus leaves (nori seaweed may be used as substitute)*
> *4 tbs roasted sesame seeds*
> *1 tsp ground black pepper*

Sauce Ingredients:
> *1 tbs (15 ml) light soy sauce*
> *1 tbs tapioca flour*
> *1 tbs (15 ml) sesame oil*

Marinate chicken in sauce ingredients for half an hour. Add sesame seeds and black pepper; mix well. Wrap each piece of chicken in pandanus leaf, and secure by tying a knot in the leaf. Heat oil on medium heat in wok. Fry chicken pieces for 5 minutes until cooked. Drain on paper towel, and serve with sweet chili sauce.

SWEET CHILI SAUCE

A great accompaniment for either of the preceding dishes, or any time you long for a spicy, tangy dipping sauce.

> *100 g coriander root, chopped finely*
> *250 g garlic, chopped*
> *7 big red chilies, finely chopped*
> *700 g palm sugar*
> *150 g white radish, sliced in thin strips*
> *375 ml vinegar*
> *1/4 tsp salt*

Put all ingredients in sauce pan, and simmer on low heat for 20 minutes until sauce is thick, stirring occasionally. Once cooked, sauce can be bottled and stored for up to one month in refrigerator.

Desserts

"ITALIAN ICE" A LA THAILAND

An easy dessert, and a soothing relief for sore throat, laryngitis, fever, and flu. A great substitute for ice cream, and an instant refresher on a hot day.

Main Ingredients:
> *coconut cream (unsweetened)*

*1 tbs palm sugar, melted in 250 ml water (raw cane sugar can
    be used as a substitute)*
shaved ice

Toppings (any or all of the following):
corn, cooked
barley, cooked
bananas, chopped
cantaloupe or honeydew melon, cubed
dates, de-pitted
raisins
taro, cooked and cubed
sweet potato, cooked and cubed
pumpkin, cooked and cubed

*Prepare small bowls of shaved ice by adding 2 tbs (30 ml) coconut cream,
1 tbs of palm sugar, water, and a pinch of salt. Top with any or all of the
toppings.*

Note: A winter variation of this dish can be made by heating coconut
milk, palm sugar, salt, and toppings, and eating warm.

SESAME LEAF SNACK

A simple and delicious treat that strengthens joints and muscles and
gives energy to the body—recommended for those suffering from bone
problems, osteoporosis, and arthritis.

sesame leaf
fresh coconut, shredded
peanuts
sesame seeds

Bundle ingredients in sesame leaf. Steam 10 minutes. Serve warm or cold.

Drinks

TONIC SHAKE

A tonic for health, strength, and vitality with a stimulating effect on the
digestion and a detoxifying effect on the body.

1 cup (approx. 150 g) pineapple
1 cup (approx. 150 g) longan
1 cup (approx. 150 g) papaya fruit
1 tsp papaya seeds
1 mandarin orange
60 ml coconut cream
60 ml fresh sugar cane juice or honey

Squeeze juice from orange and liquefy all ingredients in blender. Drink cold.

MANGO LASSI

A very popular drink in India, and increasingly so in Thailand, lassi is a delicious and refreshing nutritive tonic. The mango and rosewater in this recipe create a taste sensation and assist the yogurt in stimulating the digestive processes. Acidophilus content in yogurt is higher if it is freshly made at home.

> *250 ml plain raw milk yogurt (soy yogurt may be used as dairy substitute)*
> *125 ml water*
> *125 ml chipped or shaved ice*
> *1 mango*
> *1^1/$_2$ tbs palm sugar, cane juice, or raw unrefined sugar*
> *^{1}/$_4$ tsp rose water or 2–3 drops essential oil of rose*
> *1 tsp each chopped raw cashews and white raisins*

Combine yogurt, water, ice, mango and sugar in blender. Sprinkle rosewater on top, garnish with cashews and raisins, and serve immediately.

AVOCADO SHAKE

A tasty and unusual drink found in Southeast Asia, an avocado shake will surprise you with its sweet, fruity flavor, and it is packed with vitamins and beneficial fatty acids.

> *375 ml cup raw milk or plain soy milk*
> *125 ml cup chipped or shaved ice*
> *1 avocado*
> *1^1/$_4$ tbs palm sugar, cane juice, or raw unrefined sugar*

Combine milk, ice, avocado and sugar and in blender. Serve immediately.

Hot Juices

Thai fruit and vegetable juices are typically salty and sweet, and are frequently drunk warm. Place the ingredients in a blender with an equal

HOT JUICES AND THEIR INDICATIONS	
Fruit Juice	Indication
Tamarind	Constipation
Unripe Guava	Diarrhea
Lemon and Honey	Fever, Cold, Congestion
Carrot, Orange, Ginger and Lime	Nausea, Allergies
Tomato (with skin), Lemongrass, Black Pepper, Cayenne Pepper	Digestion

part of water, and liquefy. Strain, heat over low flame without boiling, add sugar or other sweetener to taste, if desired, and a half-teaspoon of salt per serving. You will be surprised at how delicious they are!

Herbs in Cosmetics

While most of this chapter has concerned food, some mention should be made of the traditional place of herbs in cosmetics. Herbs are commonly used cosmetically for their natural tonifying, rejuvenative, and antibacterial properties. Even today, in the most modern cities in Thailand, some of the following traditional recipes enjoy more popularity than the latest brand-name items. I recommend trying these natural recipes for a period of a few weeks, while abstaining from commercial products in order to compare results. While a few of these recipes may take some getting used to, in a short time you will easily see the benefits of using homemade natural remedies instead of the massed produced chemical alternatives. All of these preparations are 100% natural, and by using them you will lessen your exposure to unnatural chemical compounds common in today's health and beauty preparations.

In most of these recipes, I have purposely left out the proportions of the active ingredients in order to encourage experimentation. Have fun mixing your own products, and keep a log of what works (and what doesn't)!

Body Lotion (for Dry Skin)

Coconut oil and olive oil are great moisturizers. In fact, their main use in Thailand is cosmetic, and they are commonly sold at the pharmacy rather than at the grocery store! Use olive oil for moderate to dry skin and coconut for severely dry skin. Add 1 part fresh aloe gel to 2 parts oil, and apply thinly to body. Allow 20–30 minutes for the vitamins and nutrients to soak into the skin. Rinse off with warm water in the shower (don't use soap) and towel vigorously. For best results, an oil rub should follow a full-body dry-brush with natural fiber loofah or body brush.

Body Lotion (for Oily Skin)

Make the preceding oil, substituting light olive oil. In addition to aloe gel, add a splash of tamarind juice or kaffir lime juice and a dash of cider vinegar. Apply thinly and allow 20–30 minutes to soak in. The astringent action of the fruit juice in this recipe will cut through grease and cleanse the pores, while the cider vinegar helps maintain the skin's natural pH balance.

Shampoo Substitute

An effective hair wash can be made by adding 2 handfuls of eucalyptus leaves (freshly mashed with mortar and pestle) to a quart (1 liter) of cold water along with one of the following ingredients:

jasmine   *damask rose*
ylang-ylang   *champak*

Let stand overnight, strain, and use as a rinse for hair. You will have to experiment with the quantity of eucalyptus. Use smaller amounts for dry hair, more for oily. Where fresh herbs are not available, a few drops of pure essential oil may be substituted. Either mixture will keep up to 7 days if refrigerated. Eucalyptus is the cleansing agent in this shampoo, but Thai shampoos can also be made with kaffir lime, soap nut, neem, pomelo leaf, and other herbs. Try these if they are available in your area. Note that essential oils can always be substituted when fresh ingredients can not be found.

Face and Body Mist

Cold-infused flower water is also perfect as a cleansing face and body mist. Soak any fragrant flowers (such as jasmine, rose, or ylang-ylang) in cold water overnight, and strain. A standard spray-bottle is ideal to deliver an even mist to the face and body. When making mists, use distilled water for longer shelf life, and if using essential oils, be sure to use a moderate concentration to avoid irritation of face.

Hot Oil Hair Treatment

Coconut oil, almond oil, or extra virgin olive oil can give body and life to dry, brittle, or damaged hair. Mix in a splash of lime juice and mashed watermelon rind. Apply to the hair, making sure to rub the oil into the roots and scalp as well. Stand outside in direct sunlight for 10–15 minutes, allowing your hair to drink in the oil's nutrients and richness before rinsing off in the shower (but don't shampoo).

Herbal Facial

To soften skin, eliminate acne, combat wrinkles, and ease topical irritations, the Thais use powdered ginger, a natural antibacterial and skin toner. Mix 2 tbs powdered ginger with 4 tbs of either:

honey (for dry skin)   *kaffir lime juice (for oily skin)*

Stir to a paste-like consistency. Apply to the face, taking care to avoid mouth and eye areas. For best results, let the mask sit 15 minutes. While rinsing with warm water, gently scrub for a mild exfoliant.

Papaya Exfoliant

Ripe papaya is a natural exfoliant and skin-softener. Use fruit pulp, or apply the rind directly to the skin. Let stand for 15 minutes before rinsing.

Non-Alcoholic Skin Toner

Lemon juice and tamarind juice can both be used as natural astringents, are safe to apply to the face, and confer the benefits of vitamins and minerals to the skin at the same time as they cut through grease and grime. A teaspoon of cider vinegar may also be added to help maintain the natural pH balance of the skin.

Natural Antiseptic and Aftershave

Eucalyptus is one of nature's most naturally antibacterial plants. I recommend using fresh leaves, but essential oil of eucalyptus may be used as a substitute when diluted. For the first time, use at most 1 fl. oz. (30 ml) oil in 1 pint (500 ml) warm water. Try this mixture as a soothing balm after shaving, but remember that eucalyptus is a strong topical antiseptic and should not be applied to sensitive areas. A teaspoon of cider vinegar may also be added to help maintain the natural pH balance of the skin.

Lip Balm

Heat up 1 part beeswax and 3 parts coconut oil over a low flame until melted. Remove from heat and let cool in a metal or glass container. Use as necessary for dry, chapped lips, nose, and hands.

Tooth Powder

While it may seem initially strange for those of us who grew up on commercial toothpaste, natural tooth powder can be made that is just as effective, and it is 100% chemical free. The base for tooth powder is 4 parts baking soda, 1 part sea salt. Medicinal plants and oils such as neem, peppermint, cinnamon, cloves, butterfly pea, or toothbrush tree may be added, as may alum powder for treatment of tooth decay, gum disease, and abscesses.

Mouthwash and Breath Freshener

Many of the herbs in this collection may be used as a light antiseptic mouthwash for combating oral bacteria, mouth sores, and bad breath. The following herbal teas can be used as a gargle after brushing teeth.

Any combination of these may be used and may be mixed with other herbs or flowers (such as peppermint, jasmine, or lotus) for enhanced flavor:

cinnamon	cloves	eucalyptus
galangal	ginger	neem
paracress	sea salt	senna
ti	toothbrush tree	

For more information on the herbs' specific properties, refer to the individual entries in *Chapter VI*.

Homemade Tiger Balm™

A favorite topical application for soothing sore muscles. For colds, congestion, and sinusitis, apply to chest and throat. Homemade Tiger Balm™ can be made using the following ingredients:

10 drops essential oil of peppermint
10 drops essential oil of eucalyptus
5 drops essential oil of cinnamon
5 drops essential oil of clove
60 ml extra-virgin olive oil or coconut oil
15 g beeswax

Heat olive oil and beeswax in a double-boiler over low heat. Stir until wax is melted. Remove from heat. Stir in essential oils, and pour into small glass or metal containers to cool.

Note that commercial Tiger Balm™ is available in several strengths, and that you may adjust quantities of essential oils in this recipe. This balm may also be made using Vaseline or other petroleum jelly as a base for a consistency closer to Tiger Balm™.

The preceding recipe calls for essential oils, but extremely strong decoctions of fresh herbs may be used as well by following the directions below:

Combine fresh herbs in a pan with a pint (500 ml) of water; boil to reduce water. Strain. Combine liquid with oil and wax, and continue cooking over low heat until water has evaporated, making sure not to boil the oil. Remove from heat and cool in glass or metal container.

Non-toxic Insect Repellent

A perfectly safe and non-irritating insect repellent that actually works!

3 ml citronella oil	*1 ml jojoba oil*
1 ml tea tree oil	*150 ml distilled water*

Mix all ingredients in a spray bottle. Shake well before using.

Soothing Eye Drops

A remarkably easy and useful recipe:

1–2 drops aloe gel   *10 ml saline solution*

Mix well. Will keep in the refrigerator up to7 days.

HERBS IN THE HOUSEHOLD

Household products are among the most pervasive sources of harmful chemical toxins in our daily lives. The following are natural alternatives from traditional Thai kitchens:

All-Purpose Cleanser

White distilled vinegar is a cheap and natural alternative for cleaning and disinfecting counter-tops, tables, and bathroom surfaces. Dilute 1 part to 2 in water and apply with a spray-bottle. Use stronger concentration for problem areas, and add essential oils such as lavender or eucalyptus for added antibacterial action and a pleasant aroma. Pure vinegar may be used on carpets and upholstery to remove stains and odors, even from pets. Also try soaking fruits and vegetables in a light vinegar and water solution for 30 minutes to an hour before cooking to remove sediments, waxes, and pesticide residues.

Copper Tarnish Remover

Lemon and lime juice are quite effective for removing tarnish and grime from copper, silver, and other metals. Cut fresh lemons or limes into wedges, dip into salt, and rub vigorously on tarnished surfaces. For extra strength, scrub with a coconut husk or rough cloth. Rinse with water.

Aromatic Air Freshener

Put a drop or two of effervescent essential oil on a handkerchief, and drape over a lamp for two to three minutes. Small rooms will quickly be filled with a pleasant aroma without chemical perfumes or aerosol sprays, and you will benefit from the healing powers of aromatherapy at the same time. Perfect for freshening up the bathroom or creating a bit of ambiance in the bedroom. (For best results, try musky or woody scents such as patchouli or cedar.)

Natural Mothballs

For an herbal alternative to the unpleasant odor of mothballs, make a sachet with dried cedar chips, camphor, and lavender in a thin cotton cloth or cheesecloth. (A handkerchief with a few drops of essential oils may also be used.)

Mosquito-Free Zone

A popular method of keeping away mosquitoes in the Thai villages is to keep a few handfuls of fresh citronella grass under the bed. The same principle can be applied in a modern setting. Use a few drops of essential oil of citronella in a diffuser and you will sleep undisturbed.

Abrasive Cleanser

Baking soda is the perfect natural abrasive cleanser for almost any surface. Use it on stainless steel, silver, other metals, and porcelain. Works well in toilets, in ovens, and for unclogging drains. Mix 1 to 1 with salt for more abrasive action.

Windows and Glass

While not an herb, I present this option as a natural alternative and a point of interest. Newsprint is an effective cleansing agent and can be used to clean windows and other glass surfaces as well as any name-brand product, and without streaking. Spray water directly onto glass, and wipe dry with newspaper. It's that easy!

Chapter IV

Herbs in Traditional Thai Massage and Sauna

SAUNA AND STEAM BATH

The sauna or steam bath plays an important part in traditional Thai medicine. It is well known that saunas promote general health, relaxation, cleansing of the skin, and detoxification by encouraging release through the sweat pores. In the Thai tradition, specific therapeutic herbs are added to the sauna in order to enhance these effects, and in order to treat many conditions. Herbal saunas are used in treatment of respiratory diseases and infections, circulatory problems, skin disease, eye problems, sore muscles, colds, headaches, stress, and anxiety, among other ailments. Saunas are used daily by Thai mothers in the weeks after giving birth, and there are herbs that are specifically used for this purpose. A regular herbal sauna is also considered to promote longevity.

Many traditional medicine providers in Thailand—from hospitals to individual massage practitioners—have a sauna or steam bath which is either used after massage or on its own. These saunas do not necessarily have to be of the cedar-paneled variety we know in the West. One of my massage teachers in Chiang Mai built a small hot-box in her back yard from sheet metal. This "sauna" had only enough room for a single occupant, who sat on a small wooden chair. Under the chair, a single electric steamer (of the type used for steaming vegetables) provided the steam. Even more simply, I have often used a stove-top steam inhalation for colds and sinus infections. Many of the herbs listed in *Chapter VI* may be steamed or dropped in boiling water. Leaning over the pot or steamer with a towel over one's head is an ideal way to catch the aromatic vapors, although one must be careful to avoid being burnt by the hot steam or irritating the eyes.

Whatever type of inhalation therapy you are using, herbs can enhance your experience greatly. These herbs can be of any of the traditional classifications, although those of the aromatic taste naturally lend themselves to steam inhalation. You will be able to add about one ounce (30 grams) of most herbs to the steamer, but you may have to experiment with some herbs to get the perfect amount. A few herbs are extremely potent, and should be used sparingly. (For example, only a half-teaspoon of camphor is necessary for a strong effect.)

When using any type of sauna or steam bath, it is useful to remember that some herbs, such as ginger and other rhizomes, must be heated for 10–15 minutes in order to release their therapeutic benefits, while more delicate herbs, such as most flowers, are damaged by heat and are best used for no longer than 2–3 minutes. It is recommended to stagger the cooking so that all herbs reach their peak potency at the same time.

One word of caution: saunas should not be used during pregnancy or by those who are suffering from fever, hypertension, or heart disease, without consulting a doctor. Even if perfectly healthy, no one should use the sauna or steam bath for much longer than 10–15 minutes at a stretch. There is a very real possibility of overheating, and no matter how beneficial these herbs are, nausea, headache, irritated throat, and

HERBS FOR THE THAI SAUNA	
Herb	**Therapeutic Action**
Ginger, Galangal, Turmeric, Zedoary, Cassumunar Ginger, Zerumbet Ginger	General tonic for health and longevity, decongestant for colds, sinusitis, disinfectant for wounds or skin disease
Eucalyptus, Camphor Crystals, Cardamom, Thai Caper	Decongestant and bronchodilator for colds, sinusitis, bronchitis, other lung infections, and asthma; soothing of sore throats; general stimulant
Tamarind Leaf, Kaffir Lime Leaf, Soap Nut, Neem	Cleansing of skin, opening of pores
Lemongrass	Increased energy, stimulation of mind and senses
Cinnamon Bark, Ylang-Ylang Flower	Stimulation of heart
Jasmine Flower	Stimulation of heart, treatment for eye problems
Lotus Flower	Tonic for heart, circulatory system, and blood

dizziness can occur from overexposure to vapors. It is recommended to take breaks and cold showers every 10–15 minutes, and to stop immediately if you experience any discomfort.

Skin Conditioner

Before entering the sauna, one of the following skin conditioners are frequently applied directly to the skin.

Astringents for oily skin: *tamarind*   *kaffir lime juice*

Emollients for dry skin: *honey*   *powdered milk*

After finishing the sauna, rinse and towel dry, but do not use soap!

HERBAL COMPRESSES

Herbal compresses are frequently used in Thailand in conjunction with traditional massage. Herbal compresses come in two varieties, hot and cold. While cold compresses are first-aid treatments, hot compresses are frequently used to treat chronic disease.

Herbs commonly used in herbal compresses are listed in the following chart. Any or all of these herbs can be added to the compress, but typically, one from each category would be included. In addition to those listed, other therapeutic plants, such as antiparasitic or antifungal herbs, can be added to treat specific conditions. Most of the herbs listed in this book with topical uses may be added to compresses. The only

HERBS FOR COMPRESSES		
Taste	**Therapeutic Benefit**	**Example Herbs**
Hot	Stimulate energy, improve circulation, reduce congestion, and relax muscles	Ginger Root Cayenne Oil
Sour	Cleanse skin, improve skin tone, treat dermatitis or rash, disinfect acne and minor cuts, kill bacteria	Tamarind Kaffir Lime Mandarin Orange Lemon
Aromatic	Stimulate the senses, relax the mind, lessen mental disturbance and stress	Jasmine Eucalyptus Camphor Cinnamon Peppermint

exceptions would be those ingredients with a noxious odor or those that have a disagreeable effect when inhaled. Topical herbs with particular healing qualities such as antiparasitics or antifungals can be found in the compendium of herbs in *Chapter VI* and in the *Index by Application.*

Hot Compress Method

According to traditional Thai energetics, hot temperatures increase energy flow, improve circulation, relax muscles, and stimulate nerves. Applied to joints and muscles, hot compresses can soothe soreness and increase flexibility. Applied to the abdominal region, they tonify and energize internal organs, and they are used in treatment of many internal diseases.

To make a Thai herbal compress, chop or break herbs into $1/2$ inch pieces, and mix in a large bowl. Lay out sections of cheese cloth (or other thin natural fabric) of about one square foot, and scoop a fist-sized amount of the herbal mixture onto each. Bundle herbs into cheesecloth, and secure with a rubber band. (Note: if large quantities of herbs are not available, wadded rags or towels with a few drops of essential oil may be used as a substitute inside the cheesecloth bundles.)

Place bundles in an electric vegetable steamer or rice steamer. If you do not have a steamer, an acceptable substitute can be made by placing a metal colander inside a large saucepan or stock-pot. Fill the pot with water up to, but not touching, the bottom of the colander, so that herb bundles will not become soaked.

Steam bundles for 5 minutes to begin to release the beneficial oils of the herbs. Since you will not be able to stagger the cooking time, you should begin to apply steam bundles as soon as they are hot, so as not to miss the benefits of the herbs that need less cooking time.

When hot, apply bundles directly to the skin, taking care not to burn the patient. (I typically test a steamed bundle on my forearm before touching it to the patient's skin.) Steamed bundles may be dipped lightly in room-temperature olive oil or coconut oil before application in order to not burn. This also imparts the soothing and moisturizing benefits of the oil.

Exchange used bundles with hot ones from the steamer as necessary. Go through the bundles clockwise, so as to keep a rotation, and close the steamer lid in between to keep the bundles hot. (You may have to experiment a bit to get the rhythm when not using an electric steamer.) Bundles may be reused several times during the course of a massage, but you should use fresh herbs for each patient. The cheesecloth can be washed and reused.

Cold Compress

Cold compresses are used mainly for sprains, bone breaks, bruises, and other acute injuries, but may also be applied to treat headaches, fevers, and other conditions. Cold compresses are "herbal ice-packs," given immediately after an injury. According to traditional Thai medical theory, cold temperatures inhibit energy flow to the injured area, preventing energy pooling and stagnation. Cold temperatures also constrict blood vessels and cause decreased circulation, thus lessening swelling, pain, and bleeding.

It is still necessary for cold compresses to be cooked in order for the therapeutic benefits of the herbs to be released. To make cold compresses, mix the herbs, bundle them, and steam them as explained earlier. Steam for 10–15 minutes. When bundles have cooked, let them cool, and place them in the freezer. Use as you would an ice-pack. Cold compresses can be re-frozen and reused two or three times, until the herbs have been exhausted.

After applying cold compresses for 24 hours, hot compresses may be used on most injuries. Exceptions to this rule would be conditions that continue with bruising, swelling, and intense pain.

SAMPLE COMPRESS RECIPES

Choosing a harmonious combination of herbs for compresses will depend on a variety of factors, including the type of treatment necessary, the mental effects of certain aromas, and the preferences of the patient. Here are several of my favorite herbal compress recipes. (Note that you may substitute essential oils for hard-to-find herbs, although the oils will dissipate much more quickly, and you will have to re-apply often.)

ENERGY BOOST

The traditional recipe. For stimulation of mind, body, and energy. The hot herbs in this compress are penetrating and dissipating, and are typically used to soothe and relax tense, sore, pulled, or over-worked muscles; to open energy lines; and to break up congestion.

ginger root   *eucalyptus leaves*
cinnamon leaves   *kaffir lime rind and leaves*
camphor crystals

COLD-CARE COMPRESS

For clearing out congestion of the lungs, sinuses, and bronchi, apply this compress to the chest, upper back, and throat.

ginger root *eucalyptus leaves*
lemongrass stalks *cloves*
peppermint leaves

CITRUS CLEANSER AND ANTISEPTIC SKIN TREATMENT

A compress to cleanse the skin, to open the pores, and to disinfect cuts and superficial wounds.

turmeric root *eucalyptus leaves*
mandarin orange rind *lemon rind*
kaffir lime rind or leaves

AROMATHERAPY COMPRESS

The herbs in this compress have a relaxing mental effect and are useful for relieving stress, anxiety, and headaches. This recipe is also beneficial to heart patients. Apply compress to the head, face, neck, and chest for best effects. Warm bundles can also be applied over the closed eyelids.

basil leaves *peppermint leaves*
ylang-ylang flowers *jasmine flowers*

ZINGIBER COMPRESS

Especially helpful for arthritis pain, sprains, sore ligaments, and broken bones. It also soothes sore or pulled muscles and reduces pain.

ginger root *zerumbet ginger*
cassumunar ginger *galangal*
turmeric *calamus*

DRAWING COMPRESS

For drawing toxicity and negativity from the body. These herbs are cooling and work well with internal infections, blood-borne diseases, heart disease, and cancers. This compress should only be used cold, and requires no cooking.

daikon root (raw and grated)
green tea (pre-steeped in boiled water for 1 minute)
jasmine flowers

DRY SKIN HERBAL BATH

I like to use herb bundles in the bathtub, and any of the preceding recipes would work. However, the following combination of herbs has an especially soothing effect on the mind, and is great for treatment of dry or chapped skin, sunburn, and dry hair or scalp. Add 2–4 unsteamed bundles to hot bath water, allowing them to soak for 10 minutes before getting in.

papaya leaves or rind	*turmeric root*
powdered milk	*honey*
aloe gel	*chrysanthemum flowers*

Hot Herbal Pillow

Another trick with compresses is to use a hot bundle as a pillow. Lie on your back and place the compress right at the point where your neck vertebrae meet your skull. Another pillow may be placed under your lower back as well. As you lie on your back, allow your arms and legs to rest fully relaxed on the ground, and let your entire body sink into the floor. Breathe deeply and relax until the compresses have cooled.

HOT COMPRESS IN THAI MASSAGE

Thai massage is a form of manipulation therapy based on the theory of the flow of energy between specific points on the periphery of the body and the internal organs. Like other Asian massage techniques such as shiatsu and reflexology, and more recent Western developments such as myofascial release therapy, Thai massage practitioners stimulate energy lines and acupressure points on the surface of the skin to affect changes deep within the body.

Even when treating a disease or injury associated with a particular part of the body, a masseur will typically work on acupressure points throughout the body. Linked through an intricate network of energy meridians, the various acupressure points stimulate and relax the patient's mind and body, and promote the natural healing processes.

Hot compresses provide the same type of stimulation as acupressure and are often used to stimulate tender or sensitive areas that can not be massaged directly. For example, in therapy of back pain, the back may be too painful for direct acupressure, but hot herbal compress on the same points will provide similar benefits.

While it is beyond the scope of this book to discuss Thai massage or acupressure in detail, a brief note about the use of compresses for a few common ailments will be helpful. (For more information, see my book, *The Encyclopedia of Traditional Thai Yoga Massage.*) Here are a few ways in which you can use herbal compress to treat specific ailments:

- Apply a hot compress to each acupressure point in the following charts for a few minutes. (Less time if the patient experiences discomfort.)

- Begin at the extremities of the body, and work toward the center, and then work back toward the extremities to dissipate stagnant energy and stimulate new energy.

- Perform acupressure on the left side of the body first for women, and on the right side first for men. (Note that even if the symptoms appear only on one side of the body, both sides should always be massaged.)

THAI ACUPRESSURE POINTS FOR HOT COMPRESS MASSAGE

STOMACHACHE, INDIGESTION, CONSTIPATION

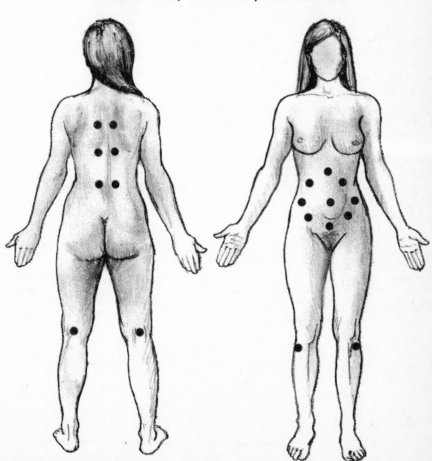

The nine acupressure points on the stomach should be treated in the following way:

1. Begin with the point in the middle.

2. Follow the contour of the large intestine by continuing clockwise around the outer points, starting and finishing with the lowest point (at 6 o'clock in the diagram).

3. Finish by treating the middle point again.

   For diarrhea, reverse this order.

LOWER BACK PAIN

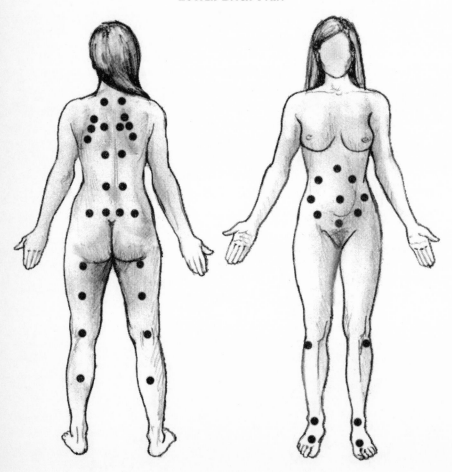

STIFF NECK, UPPER BACK PAIN, SHOULDER PAIN

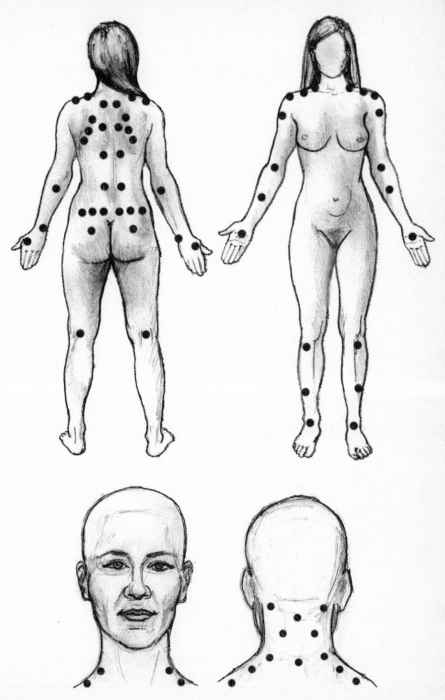

Headache, Migraine, Tension, Stress, Anxiety, Insomnia, and General Relaxation

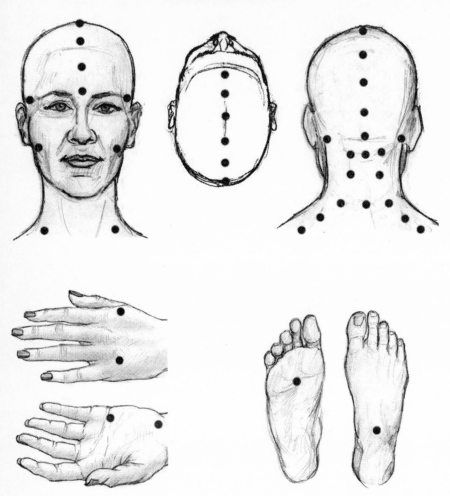

MENSTRUAL PAIN, PMS, POST-PARTUM

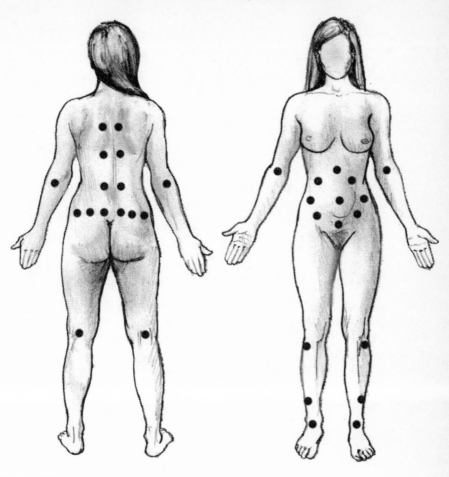

Chapter V

Herbs in Traditional Thai Medicine

METHODS OF PREPARING HERBS

Thai herbal remedies can be administered in five general ways:

Tea or Infusion

A tea, or infusion, is made by steeping herbs in hot (not boiling) water for 2–3 minutes. Generally, teas are made from delicate plant parts, such as flowers, leaves, shoots, or stems which damage easily, and therefore require a short exposure to heat for maximum benefit.

For herbal teas, the dosage often varies depending on the age, strength, and severity of illness of the patient. Unless otherwise noted, the rule of thumb is to use 1 "handful" (about an ounce or 30 grams) of fresh herb in 1 cup (250 ml) of boiled water. Halve that amount when using dried herbs. Alternatively, some teas may be made by dissolving dried powders in hot water (see *Powder* on page 65 for dosage). With any method, it is important to use enough of the herb to give the tea a strong flavor, but not so much that the consistency becomes thick.

Unless stated otherwise, teas in this collection may be drunk 1–3 times daily in 1 cup (250 ml) doses. Digestives are normally drunk after meals, while appetizers, laxatives and purgatives are taken on an empty stomach. For symptomatic relief of cough, cold, and/or sore throat, herbal teas are slowly sipped throughout the day as necessary.

Traditionally, Thai herbal teas can be taken alone or with a sweetener. Different plants are used as sweeteners depending on the particular treatment. These sweeteners are considered to be adjuvant herbs, or "helping herbs," and are listed individually later in this chapter.

Decoction

Many remedies in this pharmacopoeia are decoctions. Decoctions are similar to teas, but are made by boiling herbs in water for

10–15 minutes. This is the method of choice when using thick, fleshy, or woody herbs such as vegetables, barks, and stalks that must be cooked to release their therapeutic value. Dosage for decoctions, unless otherwise specified, is 1 "handful" (about 1 ounce or 30 grams) of herbs in 1 pint (500 ml) of water. The water will cook down, and the remedy is usually administered in a 1 cup (250 ml) dose. Sweeteners may also be added to decoctions, following the guidelines presented later in this chapter.

Powder

Many remedies that use dried seeds, nuts, or bark call for making a powder. This can be done easily by grinding with a mortar and pestle. For the modern at heart, a coffee grinder works equally well, and you may want to reserve a grinder for this particular purpose. Some powders (such as musk, for example) are almost impossible for the modern herbalist to make at home, but many of these remedies are readily available from herbal supply stores and Chinese pharmacies. (Remember, it is essential to use care when ordering herbs, especially when dealing with foreign distributors or unfamiliar products. A list of suggested retailers can be found at the end of this book.)

The usual dosage for treatment of acute conditions is 1–2 teaspoons of powder, unless otherwise specified. Use less for children, the elderly, and very weak patients. (Although in the case of nutritive tonics, larger doses may be appropriate.) Prepared powders are typically taken dry with a mouthful of lukewarm water, in a spoonful of honey, or dissolved in a cup (250 ml) of boiled water. Gelatin capsules may also be purchased at herbal supply shops.

Topical Application

Some topical applications in this collection call for the making of a powder first, which is then combined with warm water and applied to the skin as a thick paste. More often, fresh or dried herbs are mashed, bruised, or pounded with a mortar and pestle and applied as a poultice or compress. A few of the topical remedies listed here are tinctures in alcohol. These are liquid in consistency and should be applied to the skin with a cloth or cotton ball.

Steam Inhalation

Herbal remedies for the throat, lungs, and eyes are usually delivered via steam. Saunas and steam baths are commonly used in Thailand for this purpose. Alternatively, herb bundles can be steamed and placed on the chest or under the nose of a patient. (This method is best used with reclining or bed-ridden patients.) Dosage for inhaled herbs is roughly equivalent to herbal teas: about an ounce (30 grams). Inhale for no more than 15 minutes at one stretch. See *Chapter IV* for more information on steam-delivery methods.

Other Methods

Many prescriptions in this compendium are fruits and vegetables that may be readily eaten raw. When prescriptions call for cooking, these foods should be lightly steamed if not otherwise stated. Seeds are usually dry-roasted in a hot pan or wok to release beneficial oils. For the same reason, some leaves are flame-roasted by grilling over an open fire until crisp. When remedies in this collection require such preparation, it is noted in the text. Unless stated otherwise, medicinal food should be eaten alone on an empty stomach.

A Note on Essential Oils

While essential oils are not commonly used in traditional Thai medicine, they are often the most convenient and cost-efficient way to procure herbs that are rare in the West. Essential oils may be substituted for fresh or dried herbs, but only if they are genuinely pure extracts. Beware that many oils labeled "essential" are adulterated with other oils and can be toxic if taken internally. Be sure to use only reputable sources. Even with pure oils, strengths may vary from brand to brand, and you will have to experiment with dosage. Whether added to a cup of water or tea, to a poultice, or inhaled via steam, a few drops are usually all that is needed.

HERBAL MIXTURES

In the Royal Thai tradition, herbal recipes often call for a mixture of ingredients for maximum potency. The Wat Po texts list numerous remedies containing dozens of herbs in a delicate blend. While this book emphasizes herbal "simples," remedies which call for one or two plants, the art of herbal combination should nevertheless be introduced.

Herbal blending may be used to maximize the potency of a particular herb. For example, a patient who exhibits sluggish digestion could be given a combination of galangal, licorice, and aloe, to stimulate the intestines. All of these herbs have a stimulant effect on the digestion and may be used in combination. In this preparation, all of these herbs can be said to be active ingredients.

Adjuvants

Sometimes, "helping herbs" are mixed with the main medicinal herb as a complementary treatment. These herbs may have beneficial secondary effects, may lessen certain side effects of the active ingredient, or may make the taste more palatable. For example, senna is a powerful laxative used for acute constipation. However, it often causes "gripping," or intestinal cramping, when used alone. In combination with ginger, however, senna has less pronounced side effects. In this case, ginger can be said to be an adjuvant, or "helping herb," for the main ingredient, senna.

USES OF ADJUVANT HERBS	
Adjuvant Herb	**Used in...**
Aloe Cloves Ginger Licorice Turmeric Zedoary	Remedies for cough, colds, congestion, menstrual complaints, sluggish digestion, constipation, indigestion, stomachache, gas, other gastro-intestinal complaints
Cayenne	Tonics, stimulants, and remedies for constipation
Mandarin Orange	Remedies for colds, flu, low immunity, and for detoxification
Raw Milk	Nutritive tonics and strength-building remedies for emaciation and weakness
Honey	Remedies for colds, cough, sore throat, constipation, as well as in tonics
Sugar Cane Juice	Remedies for fever, sore throat, cough, congestion, bladder infections, urinary tract infections, weakness, fatigue, and emaciation
Raw, Unrefined Sugar	Remedies for fever, mouth sores, and lymph problems
Rock Sugar Palm Sugar	Remedies for fevers, colds, and sore throat
Stevia	Calorie-free sugar substitute for weight loss, hypoglycemia, and diabetes

Adjuvant herbs for specific treatments are recommended throughout the compendium of herbs in *Chapter VI*. Refer to the chart on the previous page for some commonly used adjuvant herbs and the preparations in which they are traditionally used. You may wish to add these herbs to your remedies, even when not specifically noted in the text.

Complex Combinations

In many cases, patients experience multiple symptoms which point toward multiple imbalances of the four elements. In these cases, more complex herbal preparations may be required. For example, an individual with depleted Water and excessive Fire can be given herbs for both conditions—provided that they do not interfere with each other. Referring back to the Ten Tastes Chart in *Chapter II*, the following herbs can be used for these two conditions:

	Herbs to Take	Herbs to Avoid
For Depleted Water	Oily, Salty, Sweet, Sour, Bland, Aromatic	Astringent, Bitter, Toxic, Hot
For Excessive Fire	Astringent, Sweet, Bitter, Bland, Aromatic	Oily, Salty, Toxic, Sour, Hot

As you can see, some herbs such as oily and salty herbs would help with one condition only to aggravate the other. Other herbs such as toxic and hot herbs should be avoided for both conditions. The herbs that should be prescribed in this case would be sweet, bland, and aromatic herbs, which are found in the **Herbs to Take** column for both conditions. A blend of these three tastes could work well for this patient.

Shelf-Life of Herbs

The shelf-life of herbal remedies varies depending on the substance and method of preparation. Roughly, speaking, the following may be used as a guide:

Herbal tinctures in alcohol and essential oils	Up to 2 years
Dried barks	6–8 months
Dried seeds	6–8 months
Dried roots	6 months

Dry powders	3–6 months
Fresh herbs and liquid extracts	3–5 days, up to 7 days if refrigerated

With fresh herbs and liquid extracts, it is crucial to monitor shelf-life carefully. Fresh plants loose their medicinal values rapidly, and it is important to keep in mind the length of time the herbs sat on the shelf before they were purchased. For example, "fresh" items bought at a typical supermarket may already be well past the 3–5 day period. Fresh herbs are always most effective when picked directly in a field or garden and used immediately, and most herbalists keep gardens at their homes for this purpose.

COLLECTING HERBS

As mentioned previously, Thai medicine usually involves a certain amount of spiritual and superstitious beliefs. While these topics are not covered fully in this book, it is worth pointing out that individual herbs are often associated with astrological events, numerological magic, and mythological powers. Some of this lore is mentioned in the individual entries for particular herbs, but on the whole I have attempted to leave out this material in favor of more scientific explanations which are universally acceptable.

One tidbit worth noting, however, is the correspondence between time of day and the powers of plants. The Wat Po texts explain that parts of plants should be collected at different times of day in order to maximize their potency. While this may be viewed as simple superstition, I believe there are valid reasons for some of these guidelines. For example, the Thais believe that flowers should be collected in the early morning. This also happens to be the time during which most flowers are dormant, with more fragrance and moisture than at other times of day. During the day, birds, insects, and the environment will deplete the flower's essence, and if picked for medicinal purposes, it may not have the same level of potency.

PEAK TIMES FOR HERB COLLECTION	
Time of Day	**Plant Part**
3 AM to 9 AM	Leaves, flowers, fruits, pods
9 AM to 12 PM	Branches, twigs
12 PM to 3 PM	Stem, bark, heartwood
3 PM to 9 PM	Roots
9 PM to 12 AM	Stem, bark, heartwood
12 AM to 3 AM	Branches, twigs

Special Medicinal Recipes

The following are a few of my favorite herbal concoctions from Thailand. Some are traditional recipes from ancient texts, and some are new recipes using traditional ingredients in unique combinations.

Zingiber Tea

To stimulate digestion, cure flatulence, constipation, and indigestion; to decongest lungs, sinuses, and bronchi due to cold or allergies; to encourage regular menstruation; and for a general tonic and aphrodisiac.

> 1 thumb-length ginger
> 10 ml ginseng extract
> Juice of 1/4 lemon
>
> 1 thumb-length galangal
> 1 tbs (15 ml) honey or bee pollen

Boil ginger and galangal in 4 cups (1 liter) water for 10–15 minutes. Strain. Add ginseng, lemon and honey before serving.

PMS Tea

To promote regularity in the case of blocked or infrequent menstruation; to alleviate menstrual cramping, headaches, and insomnia associated with PMS.

> 2 tsp chrysanthemum flowers
> 1 tbs fresh aloe gel
> dash black pepper
> 1/2 tbs kaffir or common lime juice to taste

Boil 2 cups (500 ml) water. Add all ingredients and steep for 2–3 minutes. Add lime juice and sweetener of your choice immediately before serving.

Digestive Tea

A gentle traditional remedy for indigestion and stomach cramps. Also great for clearing up colds, congestion, fever, and flu.

> 1 handful fresh basil leaves, flowers, and stalks
> 1 handful peppermint leaves
> 1 tsp long pepper or black peppercorns

Steep ingredients in hot water for 3–5 minutes before drinking.

IBS Tea

A soothing remedy for irritable bowel, stomach or intestinal cramps, indigestion, gastritis, and menstrual cramps. Gentle enough for children. Use honey or bee pollen as a sweetener.

2 tsp chrysanthemum flowers   4 anise stars

Steep ingredients in hot water for 3–5 minutes before drinking.

Cold-Care Tea

For colds, congestion, sinusitis, and flu. Also detoxifies, lowers fever, stimulates appetite, and promotes regular digestion.

1 handful peppermint leaves   1 handful basil leaves
2 dried eucalyptus leaves   3 tbs dried grated lemon rind

Steep ingredients in hot water for 3–5 minutes before drinking.

Antioxidant Tea

For vitamin C deficiency, detoxification, smokers, drinkers, and those who live in polluted environments.

2 oz (60 g) hibiscus flowers
20 clover blossoms
4 lemongrass stalks
1 tsp dried grated lemon or mandarin orange rind
3-inch cinnamon stick

Boil lemongrass, lemon rind, and cinnamon in 4 cups (1 liter) water 10–15 minutes. Strain. Add hibiscus and clover; steep for 2–3 minutes.

Strawberry Ginger Tea

Strawberries are in season in Northern Thailand from November through February. Strawberry tea is great for fighting colds, flu, and other minor seasonal illnesses. Served iced, it is a stimulating and refreshing summer thirst quencher.

1 thumb-length ginger
1 oz (30 g) peppermint leaves
1 oz (30 g) strawberry leaves

Boil ginger in 4 cups (1 liter) water 10–15 minutes. Strain. Add other ingredients; steep for 2–3 minutes.

Cardiac Tonic

A daily tonic for heart disease, strengthening of the heart muscle, and lowering hypertension, a traditional tea is made with equal parts of the following flowers:

lotus stamens   jasmine flowers
bulletwood flowers   ironwood flowers
sarapee flowers

Use 2 tsp at a time. Steep 2–3 minutes in hot water.

Cerebral Tonic

An Ayurvedic tonic for the brain, the senses, and the memory. Promotes immunity and longevity. Useful in cases of memory loss, debility, senility, and general loss of vitality.

1 g gotu kola
1 g loog thai bai
1 tsp honey or bee pollen

Take tea daily for up to 1 month.

Shivagakomarpaj Traditional Medicine Hospital Health & Vitality Powder

To stimulate heart, lungs, and digestion, boost energy, and heighten sexual vitality.

1 tsp lotus seed
1/2 tsp dried powdered licorice root
.1 g camphor
.1 g musk

Grind to make powder. Take 1/2 tsp daily dry or in honey, or mix with hot water.

Yaa Lueang Pid Samut

A traditional remedy for diarrhea and dysentery. Gentle enough for children and the elderly. Collect the following ingredients:

banana root   black catechu
garlic   henna leaves
nutgrass   oroxylum bark
pale catechu   pomegranate leaves
shorea bark   zedoary

Mix one part each with 6 parts turmeric. For dysentery, mix with mashed finger root and lime juice to make paste. For other diarrhea, mix with corkwood tea tree and lime juice to make paste. Form small pills from .1g of paste. Dosage 1–3 pills daily as needed while symptoms persist.

LONGEVITY TONIC

A traditional combination found in virtually any Thai market, this tea is a delicious combination of detoxifying antioxidants and tonics for longevity and vitality. For an extra immunity boost, add a slice of reishi mushroom before steeping.

1 part green tea   1 part mulberry

Steep ingredients in hot water 2–3 minutes before drinking.

TRIPHALA

Triphala is a traditional Ayurvedic remedy which is given a prominent role in Thai medicine. The Wat Po texts refer to this as the "hot season medicine," as it is prescribed for many ailments that arise at that time of year. In the Ayurvedic system, *Triphala* is one of the most prescribed compounds, valued for its laxative and tonic effects. *Triphala* is full of antioxidants and is traditionally used as a rejuvenative tonic for the elderly, and as a tonic for the brain, nervous system, memory, and senses. Use equal parts:

chebulic myrobalan   beleric myrobalan
emblic myrobalan

Powder and mix all ingredients. Take tea once daily.

TRIKATUK

The "rainy season medicine" from the Wat Po texts, this is basically a hot-herb stimulant used to treat colds and other "damp" diseases.

long pepper   ginger
black pepper

Powder and mix all ingredients. Take tea once daily.

Power Boost

This invigorating blend is a traditional energy boost with a tonic effect on the heart and circulatory system. Both ingredients increase body heat and blood flow, and for this reason are held to be powerful aphrodisiacs. Add ginseng for an extra boost. This warming brew will chase out the chills of winter, and spark your internal heat.

> *1 part safflower*   *6 parts ginger root*

Steep ingredients in hot water for 2–3 minutes before drinking.

Tea-Less Chai

A recipe from India, but one I can't resist including here. The ultimate after-dinner digestive!

> *1 thumb-length ginger*   *3-inch cinnamon stick*
> *1 tsp coriander seed, ground*   *1 tsp cardamom seed, ground*
> *1 tsp star anise seed or 3 stars*   *$^1/_2$ tsp cloves*

(Traditional chai would also include 3 tbs loose black tea.)

Boil all ingredients in 2 cups (500 ml) water for 10–15 minutes. Add 2 cups (500 ml) soy, rice, or raw milk and heat without boiling. Sweeten to taste with raw, unrefined sugar, sugar cane juice, or stevia before serving.

Chapter VI

A Compendium
of Traditional Thai
Herbal Medicine

A WARNING ABOUT DOSAGE

Traditional prescriptions are notoriously vague; "a handful" or "a pinch" is often all of the information we are given. Fortunately, with most herbal treatments, there is little danger of adverse reaction. Medicinal herbs offer a natural balance of alkaloids, which work in harmony to promote health and fight disease, while on the whole avoiding severe side effects and other adverse reactions typical of allopathic drugs.

There are some notable exceptions to this generalization in the compendium of herbs found in the next pages. Opium poppy is listed in the traditional Thai pharmacopoeia, as are several toxic plants. When a plant in this book is known to be dangerous under certain conditions, a note has been made. However, people may react to herbs in dramatically different ways, and this text can not take into account individual sensitivities and allergies. In all cases, should the patient experience nausea, dizziness, headache, diarrhea, or other adverse reactions, this should be taken as an indication that an excessive amount has been used, and less should be prescribed on subsequent occasions, or alternative herbs should be used. These warnings should be especially heeded in regard to pregnant women, children, and the elderly, who often react with greater sensitivity to herbal medicines and other drugs.

One last caveat should be noted: the claims made in this collection are based on traditional medicinal uses of these herbs. Many of the more popular herbs in this collection are well known to the West, but in the case of some of the more unusual herbs, these therapeutic claims have not been evaluated by the professional herbalist community. Although these treatments are prescribed in Thailand by reputable healers and health institutions, I have not personally tested all of the herbal prescriptions given in this collection, and I strongly emphasize that this book should not replace consultation with a competent herbalist or physician.

The compendium that follows lists herbs commonly used in traditional herbalism in Thailand. Information has been compiled from many sources—including Thai, Ayurvedic, and Western—in order to give a complete picture of the herbs and their usage in many traditions. Sources are noted in the bibliography.

Below is a sample entry, with explanation of the terminology used throughout the collection.

Note that the word "herb" is used throughout this collection to indicate a substance used by Thai herbalists and may refer to fruits, vegetables, barks, minerals, and other natural substances in addition to the more commonly held notion of an herb.

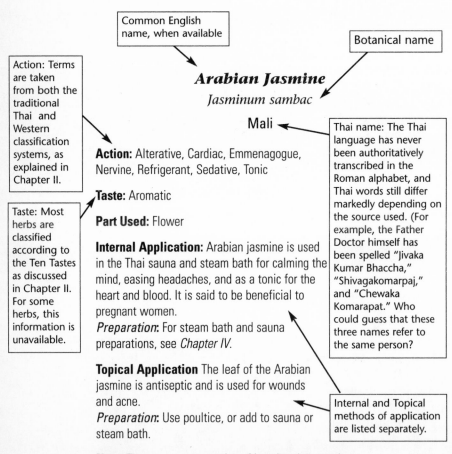

Common English name, when available

Botanical name

Action: Terms are taken from both the traditional Thai and Western classification systems, as explained in Chapter II.

Taste: Most herbs are classified according to the Ten Tastes as discussed in Chapter II. For some herbs, this information is unavailable.

Arabian Jasmine
Jasminum sambac

Mali

Thai name: The Thai language has never been authoritatively transcribed in the Roman alphabet, and Thai words still differ markedly depending on the source used. (For example, the Father Doctor himself has been spelled "Jivaka Kumar Bhaccha," "Shivagakomarpaj," and "Chewaka Komarapat." Who could guess that these three names refer to the same person?

Action: Alterative, Cardiac, Emmenagogue, Nervine, Refrigerant, Sedative, Tonic

Taste: Aromatic

Part Used: Flower

Internal Application: Arabian jasmine is used in the Thai sauna and steam bath for calming the mind, easing headaches, and as a tonic for the heart and blood. It is said to be beneficial to pregnant women.
Preparation: For steam bath and sauna preparations, see *Chapter IV.*

Topical Application The leaf of the Arabian jasmine is antiseptic and is used for wounds and acne.
Preparation: Use poultice, or add to sauna or steam bath.

Internal and Topical methods of application are listed separately.

Note: There are many species of jasmine that may be used medicinally. See also common Jasmine and Night Jasmine.

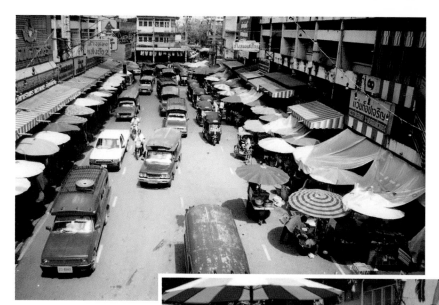

Bird's eye view of
Warorot Market,
Chiang Mai.

Drying herbs for the
sauna at the
Shivagakomarpaj
Traditional Medicine
Hospital

A colorful array of
exotic fruits are sold at
Warorot Market.

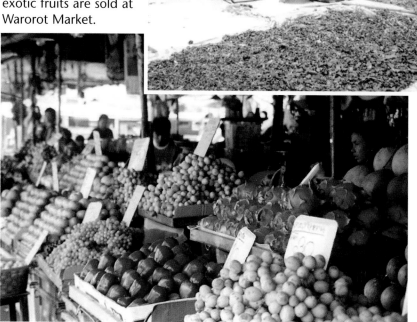

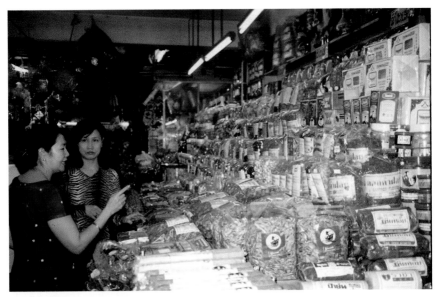

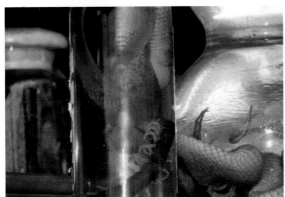

Medicinal herb markets
are a common sight in rural
Thailand.

Insects and snakes preserved
in alcohol make for potent
elixirs in the Golden Triangle
region.

The shelves of a traditional
medicine pharmacy.

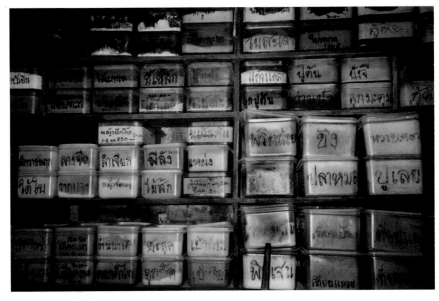

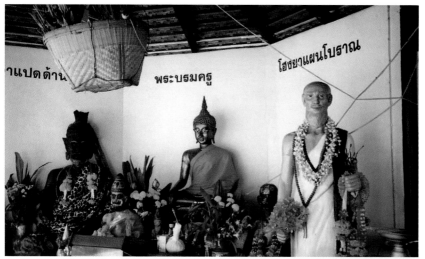

Buddhism, ancestor worship, and shamanism are mixed at the shrine to Shivagakomarpaj at the Traditional Medicine Hospital.

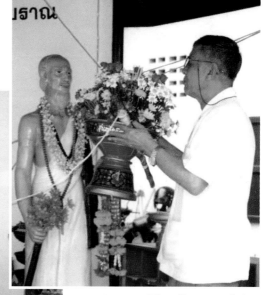

The director of the Shivagakomarpaj Traditional Medicine Hospital leads an afternoon chanting ceremony.

The Father Doctor Shivagakomarpaj at the Traditional Medicine Hospital in Chiang Mai.

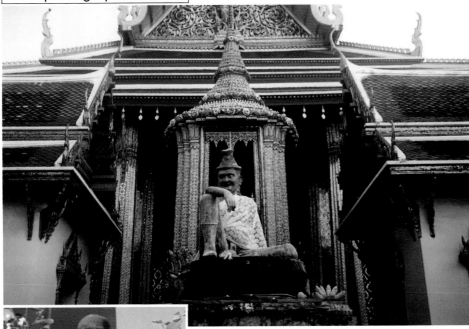

The Father Doctor watches over Wat Po,
a renowned massage school
and temple in Bangkok.

The Father Doctor is an object of veneration
at the Shivagakomarpaj Traditional Medicine
Hospital in Chiang Mai.

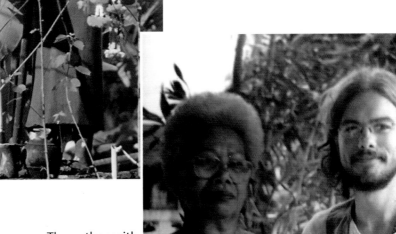

The author with
"Mama" Lek Chaiya
at her Chiang Mai
massage school.

Alexandrian Senna
Cassia acutifolia
Ma Khaam Khak

Action: Alterative, Anthelmintic, Antipyretic, Antiseptic, Cholagogue, Hepatic, Laxative, Purgative

Taste: Bitter   **Part Used:** Leaf, Pod

Internal application: Tea made from Alexandrian senna pods is a strong and effective laxative for treatment of constipation. The leaves are somewhat more gentle, and tea from the leaves is traditionally used as a mild laxative for the elderly. In smaller doses, senna stimulates the liver and encourages the production of bile, thereby aiding digestion.

Preparation: Decoction of 6–12 pods in cold water. Add 1/4 tsp ginger as adjuvant to prevent cramping. Strain; take 1–4 tbs before breakfast.

Topical application: Decoction of Alexandrian senna pods is an antiseptic. Applied topically, it is used traditionally as a treatment for bacterial and fungal skin infections. As a gargle, it is used to treat infections of the mouth, including tooth and gum disease, and mouth sores.

Preparation: Decoction as above; use as gargle and mouthwash.

Caution: Senna is not recommended for patients with hemorrhoids or for those with high levels of stress, tension, or chronic anxiety.

Note: Where C. acutifolia can not be found, the more common Western varieties, *C. Marilandica* or *C. angustifolia,* can be used.

Aloe
Aloe indica, Aloe vera
Waan Haang Jarakhe

Action: Adjuvant, Alterative, Anthelmintic, Antipyretic, Bitter Tonic, Blood Tonic, Emollient, Emmenagogue, Hepatic, Laxative, Purgative, Vulnerary

Taste: Bitter   **Part Used:** Leaf

Internal application: The Thai name for aloe translates as "alligator tail plant." Well known to the Western tradition as a bitter tonic, aloe has beneficial effects on the liver, spleen, uterus, and blood. The gel of the aloe leaves is taken internally to regulate menstruation, for detoxification, for clearing up persistent lingering illness, for liver disease, and for chronic constipation. As it is a gently detoxifying laxative, aloe is a common adjuvant in the treatment of any infectious disease. Large doses of aloe act as a purgative and can expel intestinal worms and other parasites. The Wat Po texts list aloe in recipes for parasites, vomiting, diarrhea, dysentery, constipation, mucous in the digestive tract, flatulence, fever, blood in breast milk, and infected or stagnant blood. It is used by Hill-Tribes to combat epilepsy, seizures, and rabies.

Preparation: Incise fresh mature leaves to extract gel. Take 2 tbs gel mixed with liquefied palm sugar or 1 cup (250 ml) sweet fruit juice 1–3 times daily. Or make tea from dried aloe leaves.

Topical application: Thai tradition holds that a dab of aloe gel on each temple is a great cure for tension headaches. Aloe gel is also mentioned in the Wat Po texts as a topical remedy for convulsions, tetanus, backache, boils, swelling, and tendinitis. It is commonly used topically in Eastern and Western herbalism to soothe burns, cuts, herpes, eczema, and other skin irritations. Aloe can be used in hot or cold compresses.

Preparation: Incise fresh mature leaves to extract gel. Apply topically to affected area frequently. For compresses, see *Chapter IV.*

Alum Powder
Saansom

Action: Astringent, Antiparasitic, Antiseptic

Taste: Sour	**Part Used:** Alum powder is a white crystalline salt derived from aluminum sulfate.

Internal Application: Alum powder is an antibacterial for infections of the ear, bladder, or eye. An effective astringent, it also is used to treat hemorrhoids, diarrhea, and internal bleeding.

Preparation: Take 1 tsp alum powder in hot water daily.

Topical Application: Alum powder is added to toothpaste or tooth powder to fight tooth decay and to strengthen unhealthy or loose teeth. It may be used on the skin for rashes, eczema, itching, scabies, ringworm, and other skin parasites.

Preparation: Apply powder directly to teeth with toothbrush. Rinse.

Alumina Clay

Action: Antipruritic, Astringent

Taste: Bland	**Part Used:** A white powdered clay derived from bauxite or aluminum oxide.

Topical Application: Alumina clay is applied topically to soothe skin rashes, hives, insect bites, and irritations.

Preparation: Mix clay with warm water; apply to affected areas as needed.

Angelica
Angelica archangelica
Kot Hua Bua

Action: Analgesic, Antirheumatic, Antispasmodic, Appetizer, Carminative, Diaphoretic, Emmenagogue, Expectorant, Stimulant, Stomachic, Tonic

Taste: Hot   **Part Used:** Root, Seed, Rhizome

Internal Application: Angelica is beneficial for any type of pre-menstrual symptoms, including cramps, headaches, bloat, and muscle spasms. It is also effective in promoting regular menstruation when blocked. Angelica is used as a cold remedy and against flu, fever, and generally low energy and low immunity. In small doses, it also stimulates the appetite.

Preparation: Decoction

Topical Application: Angelica is applied topically to control itching and to help heal wounds and cuts. It also may be applied with hot compress over arthritic joints to control pain.

Preparation: Mash angelica with mortar and pestle. Apply with poultice or hot compress.

Arabian Jasmine
Jasminum sambac
Mali

Action: Alterative, Blood Tonic, Cardiac, Emmenagogue, Female Tonic, Nervine, Refrigerant, Sedative, Tonic

Taste: Aromatic   **Part Used:** Flower

Internal Application: Arabian jasmine is used in the Thai sauna and steam bath for calming the mind, easing headaches, and as a tonic for the heart and blood. It is said to be especially beneficial to pregnant women.

Preparation: For steam bath and sauna preparations, see *Chapter IV.*

Topical Application: The leaf of the Arabian jasmine is antiseptic and is used for wounds and acne.

Preparation: Use poultice, or add to sauna or steam bath.

Note: There are many species of jasmine that may be used medicinally. See also Common Jasmine, and Night Jasmine.

Asafoetida
Ferula foetida, Ferula asafoetida

Action: Analgesic, Anthelmintic, Antirheumatic, Antiseptic, Antispasmodic, Aphrodisiac, Carminative, Digestive, Expectorant, Laxative, Nervine, Purgative, Sedative, Stimulant, Stomachic

Taste: Hot   **Part Used:** A resin is extracted by incising the roots of the fresh plants

Internal Application: As a hot herb, asafoetida is used in Thai medicine to stimulate digestion and to help cases of flatulence, indigestion, and constipation. Its expectorant action makes it ideal to fight colds, congestion, and asthma. A daily dose of asafoetida is reputed to be a tonic for the brain and senses, and is also recommended to counter arthritis. In large doses, it is a purgative used to expel intestinal worms.

Preparation: Take decoction of 1 tsp resin or 1 gram powder in 1 pint (500 ml) hot water daily. Use ginger as an adjuvant to lessen side effects and enhance the flavor of this treatment.

Topical Application: Topically, a poultice of asafoetida may be used to soothe arthritis and other joint pain.

Preparation: Make thick paste by adding warm water to resin; apply to affected areas.

Bael
Aegle marmelos
Matoom

Action: Antiseptic, Astringent, Carminative, Expectorant, Stimulant, Stomachic

Taste: Hot   **Part Used:** Fruit, Leaf

Internal Application: The ripe bael fruit is traditionally used as a decongestant for the common cold, especially when there is excessive congestion of the lungs, as well as for tuberculosis and typhoid fever. It is also prescribed for any type of disorder of the intestines, including diarrhea, constipation, flatulence, and dysentery. Bael fruit is used for its stimulating properties in cases of exhaustion and convalescence from chronic disease or injury, but it is said to inhibit sexual energy, and is for that reason drunk by monks at many monasteries. Unripe bael fruit is an astringent, used as an antidiarrheal and as a daily tonic. Juice from the crushed leaves of the bael is given for respiratory infections, and decoction of the stem is said to be a useful antimalarial.

Preparation: Fruit is eaten raw or is sliced, dried, and boiled to make a decoction.

Topical Application: Bael leaves may be used topically as an antibacterial and antifungal for skin infections or wounds.

Preparation: Mash a handful of leaves with mortar and pestle, adding water to make a paste. Apply to affected areas.

Baking Soda

Action: Antacid, Antipruritic

Taste: Salty   **Part Used:** Baking Soda is powdered
                                    sodium bicarbonate.

Internal Application: In the West, we typically use baking soda as a treatment for hyperacidity and indigestion. In addition to this usage, Thai herbalists recommend a teaspoon of baking soda in a glass of warm water as a detoxifying cleanser for stomach, intestines, kidneys, and bladder.

Preparation: Take one tsp in lukewarm water.

Topical Application: Baking soda is useful topically on insect bites and stings (especially bee and wasp), rashes, itchiness, and skin irritations. Due to its cleansing and whitening action, it is also a common ingredient in toothpaste and tooth powder (see *Chapter III* for tooth powder recipe).

Preparation: Mix with warm water to make paste. Apply to skin as needed.

Banana
Musa sapientum
Kluai

Action: Astringent, Demulcent, Diuretic, Nutritive Tonic, Stomachic

Taste: Bland　　　　　　　　**Part Used:** Fruit, Root, Sap

Internal Application: There are a 28 official species of bananas in Thailand, with marked differences in size, shape, and flavor. Each has a different name in Thai, although "kluai" is useful as a general term. Some bananas are green when ripe, some are pink, others are mottled brown, and according to traditional Thai cuisine, some are best in coconut milk, some are best raw, and some are only eaten soaked in honey and dried. The flowers of the banana plant are similar in texture to cabbage and are eaten in salads or in curries. The rest of the plant is utilized as well: the roots of the banana plant are converted into mulch, the fibers are woven into twine, and the leaves are used as plates and containers. A common method of cooking is to wrap ingredients such as rice, beans, fish, or vegetables in a banana leaf before grilling or steaming. The banana is also a source of wine, vinegar, cloth dye, and flour. Pureed banana is a popular baby food, and batter-fried bananas are a favorite street-stall snack.

A banana, in botanical terms, is actually a berry. The fruit is high in vitamins A and C, potassium, and carbohydrates, and therefore the ripe fruits are useful for emaciation and wasting diseases. The unripe banana is used traditionally as a stomachic to treat diarrhea and peptic ulcers. The ripe fruit is demulcent, the roots are diuretic, and the sap of the stem is astringent.

Preparation: Eat 1–2 unripe fruits. Raw fruit may also be dried and ground to make powder. Dosage is 3–4 tbs of powder mixed with 1–2 tbs honey. Take 4 times daily, with meals and before bed. Note that this remedy may cause flatulence. Other methods of preparation include decoction of root and sap.

Beleric Myrobalan
Terminalia belerica
Samoh Phipheg

Action: Anthelmintic, Antiseptic, Antitussive, Astringent, Digestive, Expectorant, Laxative, Pectoral Tonic

Taste: Astringent　　　　　　　　**Part Used:** Fruit

Internal Application: The beleric myrobalan fruit is a very important herb in the Ayurvedic tradition, and consequently, in the Royal Thai tradition as well. It is considered to be a rejuvenative tonic, a tonic for the lungs, larynx, throat, bronchi, digestive system, and eyes, and to encourage hair growth. The ripe fruit is an astringent to treat diarrhea, dysentery, and other intestinal parasites, but the unripe fruit is a strong laxative, which will correct constipation. Unripe beleric myrobalan fruit corrects all types of stones, parasites, and blockage in the digestive, urinary, and respiratory tracts. It is also an expectorant used to treat cough, sore throat, laryngitis, and bronchitis.

Preparation: Take 250 mg to 1 g powdered dried fruit with honey.

Topical Application: Decoction of beleric myrobalan is a topical antiseptic.

Note: This herb is often combined with chebulic myrobalan and emblic myrobalan, found elsewhere in this collection. (See Triphala in *Special Medicinal Recipes, Chapter V,* for more information on this combination.)

Betel Leaf
Piper betel
Phlu

Action: Antiparasitic, Antipruritic, Antiseptic, Bronchodilator, Expectorant, Stimulant

Taste: Hot   **Part Used:** Leaf

Topical Application: The leaf of the Piper betel is commonly used to wrap a small amount of betel nut (Areca catechu), an addictive stimulant nut chewed by many throughout South Asia. The betel leaf is used topically as an antibacterial and as a treatment for allergic hives, itching, ringworm, and skin parasites. Betel leaf applied topically to the chest acts as a decongestant and bronchodilator and is successfully used in cases of congestion, difficult respiration, asthma, and diphtheria.

Preparation: Mash 3–4 fresh leaves with mortar and pestle, adding alcohol to make a paste. Apply to affected areas 4 times daily for 3–5 weeks. For respiratory ailments, this poultice may be applied liberally to chest and throat as needed while symptoms persist.

Bitter Gourd, Bitter Melon, Balsam Pear
Momordica charantia
Mala

Action: Alterative, Anthelmintic, Antioxidant, Antipyretic, Bitter Tonic, Blood Tonic, Carminative, Cholagogue, Digestive, Hepatic, Laxative, Stomachic

Taste: Bitter   **Part Used:** Fruit, Leaf

Internal Application: Bitter gourd works powerfully to detoxify the blood and colon. This fruit is commonly used in rural Thailand to fight HIV-AIDS, hepatitis, and cancer, as well as other systemic diseases. It has particularly beneficial effects on diseases of the liver, spleen, and pancreas. The juice of the vegetable is a laxative and antipyretic. Eaten daily as a bitter tonic, steamed bitter gourds are routinely suggested for the elderly, diabetics, hypoglycemics, and those with chronic disease or illness. It has also been shown to increase insulin production and to have anti-carcinogen properties. As it encourages proper digestion, bitter gourd is recommended for sluggish digestion, dysentery, chronic constipation, and flatulence. It is also reputed to be beneficial for poor eyesight and is high in the antioxidant vitamins A and C. Bitter gourd is listed in the Wat Po texts as an appetizer, purgative, anthelmintic, and as a cure for leprosy. It appears in treatments for fever, infections, menstrual problems, hemorrhoids, and constipation.

Preparation: Eat vegetable lightly steamed, preferably with chili sauce. Or drink fresh juice from raw vegetable.

Topical Application: The juice of the bitter gourd can be used topically on the skin and in the mouth as an antiseptic. The leaves are mentioned in the Wat Po texts in topical remedies for tendinitis, swellings, infections, and headaches.

Preparation: Liquefy fresh vegetable in blender or juicer.

Black Bean
Castanospormum australe
Tua Pum

Action: Antirheumatic, Diuretic

Taste: Oily   **Part Used:** Bean, Pod

Internal Application: Black beans are used traditionally in dietary regimes for arthritis and other joint problems. Black beans also have been shown to help control blood sugar, and thus are recommended for diabetics and hypoglycemics. In Western herbalism, the pod of the plant is used for its diuretic properties in kidney or bladder disorders.

Preparation: Eat beans cooked. Make tea from fresh or dried bean pod.

Black Pepper
Piper nigrum
Prik Thai Dam

Action: Antipyretic, Carminative, Digestive, Expectorant, Stimulant, Stomachic

Taste: Hot   **Part Used:** Fruit

Internal Application: The fruit of the black pepper, also known as the peppercorn, turns red when it is ripe. The riper the seed, the more potent the medicinal effects, and fresh red seeds are the only type commonly used by herbalists. It is said in Thailand, however, that the most medicinal peppercorns are those that are found in bird droppings. Black pepper is a hot herb used traditionally for treating colds, congestion, sore throat, sinusitis, and fever. Like most hot herbs, it is also a powerful digestion stimulant. It is also used to treat chronic coldness, temporary mild paralysis (such as Bell's Palsy syndrome), and for general stimulation of the Fire element.

Preparation: Make tea from 1 tsp dried peppercorn in 1 cup (250 ml) water. Black pepper is commonly used with basil as a cold remedy, and is usually accompanied by honey as an adjuvant. (See *Special Medicinal Recipes, Chapter V.*)

Caution: Black pepper may be slightly poisonous if excessive doses are taken frequently.

Blue Crab, Horseshoe Crab
Putalay

Action: Female Tonic, Nutritive Tonic

Taste: Salty   **Part Used:** Claw of *Scylla serrata,* a sea-crab

Internal Application: The meat of the blue crab is prized by traditional Thai healers for its tonic properties. It is typically given to children to protect from common childhood diseases and to women for tonification of the uterus and other female reproductive organs after pregnancy.

Preparation: Eat steamed.

Note: The field-crab, *Paratelphusa sexpunctatum,* which lives in inland rice paddies, is often substituted by those who live far from the sea.

Bulletwood
Mimusops elengi
Mak sa koun

Action: Antipyretic, Antirheumatic, Cardiac, Female Tonic, Sedative

Taste: Aromatic   **Part Used:** Flower, Wood

Internal Application: The bulletwood flower, like many herbs with aromatic taste, is taken either as tea or used in the sauna. It is administered through inhalation to treat arthritis, heart disease, as well as to calm anxiety, stress, and panic attacks. The tea is used to treat fevers, sore throat, and muscular pain. Tea made from the wood is considered to be a tonic for the heart and circulatory system, and a tonic for pregnancy, especially when the wood is infected by a particular fungus which gives the bark a mottled appearance. Decoction of the stem bark is used as a gargle for gingivitis.

Preparation: Make tea from dried flowers or decoction from wood.

Butterfly Pea, Blue Pea
Clitorea ternatea
Aan Chan

Action: Antirheumatic, Diuretic, Laxative, Stomachic   **Part Used:** Seed, Root

Internal Application: The butterfly pea seed is used to treat constipation and to soothe stomach pains and cramps. The root has similar properties but is also a diuretic and an antirheumatic. The decoction is dropped into the eyes to treat poor vision and is added to toothpaste or powder to treat toothache. This herb is also a hair tonic, used to treat baldness and falling hair.

Preparation: Tea or powder.

Burr Bush
Triumfetta rhomboidea
Seng

Action: Antipyretic, Stomachic   **Part Used:** Whole plant

Internal Application: The burr bush is used by Hill-Tribes to treat stomachache, indigestion, and to treat fever during menstruation.

Preparation: Decoction

Calamus, Sweet Sedge, Sweet Flag, Myrtlegrass
Acorus calamus
Waan nam

Action: Antirheumatic, Antispasmodic, Antitussive, Aphrodisiac, Carminative, Diaphoretic, Emetic, Emmenagogue, Expectorant, Nervine, Stimulant, Stomachic, Tonic

Taste: Hot   **Part Used:**   Rhizome

Internal Application: Calamus is a stomachic traditionally used to treat indigestion, heartburn, gastritis, and hyperacidity, as well as to encourage appetite. Like most hot herbs, it is an effective cold cure and decongestant. It is used particularly against cough, lung congestion, asthma, sinusitis, and fever. Calamus is considered to be a beneficial tonic and stimulant for the nervous system, especially the senses and the brain. Ayurvedic tradition prescribes calamus tea for sufferers of typhoid, epilepsy, deafness, and arthritis, and to help expel kidney stones. Taken daily, calamus is said to enhance memory and sexual energy. In Western herbalism, smokers are told to chew the fresh rhizome in order to cause a slight bit of nausea which aids in quitting smoking.

Preparation: Take decoction once daily. Use ginger as an adjuvant with calamus preparations.

Topical Application: Calamus is traditionally applied topically over painful joints and fractured or broken bones.

Preparation: Mash root; apply locally to affected area with poultice or hot compress.

Caution: Calamus should not be used in cases of bleeding disorders, as it thins the blood.

Camphor
Cinnamonum camphora
Ga ra boon

Action: Analgesic, Anti-inflammatory, Antirheumatic, Antiseptic, Antispasmodic, Antitussive, Bronchodilator, Cardiac, Diaphoretic, Emmenagogue, Expectorant, Nervine, Pectoral, Sedative, Stimulant

Taste: Hot and Aromatic   **Part Used:**   Crystals derived from the gum of the tree trunk

Internal Application: Camphor is used in nearly all of the religious ceremonies in India and carries a spiritual connotation throughout the rest of Asia as well. As it burns without leaving any ash, it is commonly considered to be a metaphor for the Enlightened mind, which vanishes into Nirvana without a trace. Camphor crystals are a common ingredient in most Thai saunas, from the traditional hospitals to the modern health clubs.

Camphor is a bronchodilator and a decongestant, and is inhaled to treat colds, congestion, sore throat, cough, bronchitis, and sinusitis. Inhalation of camphor is also beneficial for irregular or blocked menstruation, eye infections, fevers, typhoid, and lung infections. Camphor crystals stimulate the brain, heart, and circulation, but paradoxically have a calmative effect on stress, anxiety, and insomnia. Camphor is therefore listed both as a calmative and a stimulant, and it is used both internally and externally in small quantities for both purposes. The wood of the camphor tree is used as an expectorant and carminative.

Preparation: For more information on inhalation by steam bath or sauna, see *Chapter IV.* Only a sprinkle of camphor crystals is necessary to experience the stimulating effects. Dosage for sauna, steam bath, or compress is $^1/_2$ – 1 tsp. Internal dosage is no more than .05 grams.

Topical Application: Camphor crystals are used topically as an anti-inflammatory for arthritis, sprains, and muscle pain, and as an antiseptic and analgesic on mild cuts, insect bites, and skin infections.

Preparation: Apply crystals topically with hot towel or compress.

Caution: In excessive doses, camphor is a narcotic poison and overdose may cause convulsions.

Candelabra Bush, Ringworm Bush,
Cassia alata, Senna alata
Chumet Thet

Action: Antiparasitic, Antiseptic, Diuretic, Laxative

Taste: Bitter **Part Used:** Leaf, Flower

Internal Application: The candelabra bush, like other cassias, is used as a laxative. It is mentioned in the Wat Po texts as a cure for constipation, flatulence, diarrhea caused by intestinal parasites, and blood or mucous in the stools. It is said that it should be "powdered together with zedoary and dusted on the body of a child who is difficult to rear, in order to prevent illness."

Preparation: Eat two or three fresh flower clusters, lightly steamed, with chili sauce. Or flame-roast 12–15 dried leaves. Make decoction; take before breakfast or at bedtime. For tapeworms or other intestinal parasites, use the "Five Parts" remedy—trunk, root, fruit, flowers, and leaves powdered together.

Topical Application: The leaves of the candelabra bush are used topically as an antiseptic and antiparasitic for treatment of ringworm, fungal and bacterial skin infections, and wounds.

Preparation: Bruise or crush fresh leaves with mortar and pestle, combining with alcohol or lime juice to make paste. Apply topically to affected areas twice daily as a poultice or hot compress. The decoction described above may also be used topically.

Note: Note that candelabra bush leaves may cause nausea and vomiting if the leaves are not fully roasted, and may cause cramping. This plant should not be used for children or patients with inflammatory bowel diseases. Overdose may cause damage to kidneys. Prolonged use may cause chronic diarrhea.

Cardamom
Amomum krervanh, Amomum xanthioides, Amomum uliginosum
Krawaan *(Amomum krervanh)*, Wan Sao Lowng *(Amomum xanthioides)*, Reo krawaan *(Amomum uliginosum)*

Action: Antitussive, Carminative, Diaphoretic, Expectorant, Stimulant, Stomachic

Taste: Hot   **Part Used:** Seed

Internal Application: Cardamom is known for its stimulating qualities and soothing effects on the gastrointestinal system. The tea is taken all over the world for flatulence, bloated stomach, sluggish digestion, irritable bowel syndrome, and gastritis. In Thailand, Siamese cardamom and bastard cardamom are used to ease stomach pain and cramping associated with gastritis and indigestion. Cardamom is also widely used as a cough suppressant, as well as to treat colds, bronchitis, asthma, and laryngitis.

Preparation: Make powder from dried seeds. Take 2 tsps in warm water or in herbal tea after meals. For cough, drink tea or suck on whole seeds.

Note: Where these varieties of cardamom are not available, common cardamom *(Elettaria cardamom)*, may be used.

Caricature Plant, Golden Leaves
Graptophyllum pictum

Action: Antipyretic, Blood Tonic, Hepatic, Tonic

Taste: Bland   **Part Used:** Leaf

Internal Application: The caricature plant is used traditionally to detoxify the system, especially in cases of fever, chronic thirst, measles, or food poisoning. It is considered to be a tonic and detoxifying agent for the liver.

Preparation: Tea. Drink 1–3 times daily.

Cashew
Anacardium occidental
Ma-muang-him-ma-pa, Tua cashew

Action: Expectorant, Nutritive Tonic

Taste: Oily   **Part Used:** Nut, Leaf, Bark, Flower

Internal Application: Cashew nuts are a common ingredient in Thai appetizers and desserts, and are often stir-fried with chicken and sweet and sour sauce. As with most oily herbs, cashews nuts are recommended by traditional herbalists as a part of the daily diet for those suffering from skin or bone problems, chronic skin infections, dry skin, or frequent allergic rashes. As it is high in caloric energy, protein, and potassium, the cashew nut is a nutritive tonic that gives increased energy and strength, and is therefore beneficial in cases of emaciation, low immunity, low energy, and chronic disease. The young shoots and leaves are eaten raw or in soups, and are expectorants. Decoction of the bark or flower is used to treat diarrhea and dysentery.

Cassod Tree, Siamese Cassia
Cassia siamea
Kee Lek

Action: Antioxidant, Antipyretic, Appetizer, Diuretic, Laxative, Sedative, Stomachic, Tonic

Taste: Bitter   **Part Used:** Leaf, Shoot, Flower, Wood

Internal Application: The young leaves and flower buds of the cassod tree are often eaten in curries and soups. Medicinally, decoction of the flower or the heartwood is used as a calmative for cases of anxiety, stress, and nervousness. The wood is also used to reduce fever. The flowers and leaves of the cassod tree are used to treat insomnia and as a general tonic high in vitamins A and C. Both are effective laxatives, stimulating digestion and promoting appetite.

Preparation: Decoction from 2–3 handfuls of young shoots, leaves, and/or wood boiled in water with a pinch of salt. Take before bed. For insomnia, a tincture in alcohol is made by soaking shoots and flowers in alcohol for 7 days. Stir frequently. Strain, and take 1–2 tsps at bedtime.

Cassumunar Ginger
Zingiber cassumunar
Phrai

Action: Anti-inflammatory, Astringent, Bronchodilator, Carminative, Emmenagogue, Laxative, Vulnerary

Taste: Hot   **Part Used:** Rhizome

Internal Application: Juice squeezed from the fresh cassumunar rhizome is taken with salt for indigestion, dysentery, diarrhea, inflammation of the intestine, and injury to internal organs. It acts as an emmenagogue, as well as a bronchodilator for treatment of asthma. Some Hill-Tribes use cassumunar ginger to help new mothers recover after delivery.

Preparation: Mash 1 thumb-length cassumunar ginger rhizome with water to make paste. Strain; mix with 1 tbs salt. Drink up to 3 times daily.

Topical Application: Cassumunar ginger is used topically to soothe contusions, sprains, and inflammations of joints and ligaments. Like common ginger, it is also used topically as an antiseptic for wounds, cuts, and skin infections. Mixed with alcohol, it is an effective mosquito repellent.

Preparation: Mash plant with mortar and pestle; add a pinch of salt, and enough water to make a paste. Apply topically to affected areas. Cassumunar ginger is a useful ingredient for hot or cold compresses (see *Chapter IV* for more information).

Castor Oil Plant
Ricinus communis
Lahung

Action: Adjuvant, Diuretic, Galactogogue, Laxative

Part Used: Oil pressed from Seed, Leaf

Internal Application: Castor oil is a gentle laxative used in Thailand mainly for the elderly and children, or as an adjuvant to other laxative or purgative remedies. Decoction of the leaf is used to stimulate breast-milk production and to increase urine to aid in expelling kidney and bladder stones and infections. The castor oil plant is used by Hill-Tribes for treatment of indigestion, ear problems, kidney disease, and post-partum recovery.

Preparation: Castor oil can be bought over the counter in most Western countries. Follow directions on packaging.

Topical Application: Castor oil is applied topically to clean wounds, infections, itching, dermatitis, rashes, inflammation, and over broken bones to speed healing.

Note: Use only cold-expressed castor oil internally. Hot-expressed oil is toxic.

Catechu
Acacia catechu
Seesiat

Action: Antiemetic, Astringent, Purgative

Taste: Astringent   **Part Used:** Resin

Internal Application: Catechu resin, known in Thai as "seesiat lao," is an ingredient in the stimulant betel nut preparations chewed in many South Asian countries. The wood is also used for dying cloth. Medicinally, it is used as an astringent and is most often used for cases of diarrhea. Catechu is also taken in larger doses as a purgative in cases of intestinal parasites, food poisoning, and allergic reactions to food including hives and nausea.

Preparation: For diarrhea, make tea from 1/2 tsp dried powdered resin in a cup (250 ml) of hot water. Drink 3 times daily before meals while symptoms persist. For purgative effect, simmer resin in water to make thick paste. Take 1 tsp paste in hot water.

Topical Application: As an astringent herb, catechu resin is frequently used topically to counteract boils, sores, skin ulcers, and infections

Preparation: Apply dried powdered resin to affected areas.

Cat's Whisker
Orthosiphon aristatus
Ya Huad Maew

Action: Diuretic   **Part Used:** Whole plant

Internal Application: As a diuretic, cat's whisker is used to treat kidney disease, gallstones, and gout. It decreases the levels of uric acid and lowers cholesterol in the blood, and is said to be a tonic for the kidneys.

Preparation: Make tea from 4 g dried powdered plant and 1 cup (250 ml) water. Sip all day long.

Topical Application: The whole plant is used topically to treat muscle pain.

Preparation: Bruise plant with mortar and pestle; make poultice. Or use in hot herbal compress.

Caution: Due to high potassium content, this herb may be dangerous for patients with heart disease.

Cayenne
Capsicum frutescens
Prik kheenuu

Action: Alterative, Anthelmintic, Antioxidant, Antiseptic, Cardiac, Carminative, Diaphoretic, Expectorant, Stimulant, Stomachic, Tonic

Taste: Hot   **Part Used:** Fruit, Leaf

Internal Application: As a hot herb, the fruit of the cayenne pepper is useful in cases of colds, flu, and congestion. A stimulant of digestion, it relieves constipation, indigestion, intestinal cramps, irritable bowel, and gastritis, and tends to increase appetite. Cayenne is a circulatory stimulant, used to treat low blood pressure, fainting, and circulatory deficiency. As an antioxidant rich in vitamins A and C, it is useful as a general tonic and detoxifier, and may be used as an adjuvant herb in preparations to boost immunity.

Preparation: Eat chili as a condiment with food. (See recipe for chili sauce in *Chapter III.*) Cayenne leaves or juice of the leaves may be added to soups or curries.

Topical Application: Essential oil of cayenne is frequently used in hot herbal compresses to relax tense muscles. It increases blood supply to skin and mucous membranes.

Preparation: See *Chapter IV.*

Caution: Do not use on sensitive skin. Topical application should be of cayenne oil, not the fresh fruits, and should be of low dosage to prevent irritation or blistering of skin. If any irritation results from topical or internal application of cayenne, discontinue use.

Champaca, Champak, Michelia
Michelia champaca, Michelia alba
Champee

Action: Antiemetic, Antipyretic, Blood Tonic, Cardiac, Diuretic, Nervine, Stimulant, Tonic

Taste: Aromatic   **Part Used:** Whole plant

Internal Application: Tea from the champaca flower, like many aromatic herbs, is used to treat fever, chronic fatigue, and low immunity. It is also prescribed traditionally as a tonic for the heart, the nervous system, and the blood. Both the flower and the fruit are diuretic, antiemetic, antipyretic, and are considered to be general tonics for the four elements. The leaf is used for neural disorders, the bark of the stem is antipyretic, and the wood is a menstrual tonic.

Preparation: Tea or decoction.

Topical Application: Decoction of the champaca flower is applied to the temples to relieve headache. Decoction of the dried ground root in milk is applied to abscesses.

Chebulic Myrobalan
Terminalia chebula
Samoh Thai

Action: Anthelmintic, Antipyretic, Antitumor, Antitussive, Astringent, Blood Tonic, Demulcent, Expectorant, Hemostatic, Laxative, Nervine, Tonic

Taste: Astringent   **Part Used:** Fruit

Internal Application: The chebulic myrobalan fruit is a very important herb in the Ayurvedic tradition, and consequently, in the Royal Thai tradition as well. The unripe fruit is a common detoxifying remedy for fever, parasitic infections, spleen disorders, jaundice, skin disease, and allergic reactions of the skin. Chebulic myrobalan corrects digestive disorders and can be used for constipation, diarrhea, dysentery, and intestinal parasites. It also has a beneficial effect on the nervous system, nervous disorders, and cancerous tumors. It is an expectorant used for colds, congestion, cough, asthma, bronchitis, and laryngitis, and an astringent used to halt blood or mucous in stool, sputum, or vaginal discharge. The ripe fruit is astringent, demulcent, and antidiarrheal.

Preparation: Eat fruit ripe or unripe.

Note: This herb is often combined with beleric myrobalan and emblic myrobalan, found elsewhere in this collection. (See Triphala in *Special Medicinal Recipes, Chapter V,* for more information on this combination.)

Chinese Chive
Allium tuberosum
Kui Chaai

Action: Anthelmintic, Diuretic, Emmenagogue, Galactogogue

Taste: Hot   **Part Used:** Leaf, Stem, Seed

Internal Application: The Chinese chive is primarily used traditionally to increase the production of urine in order to treat kidney or bladder stones, dysuria (insufficient or painful urination), and gonorrhea. The leaves of the Chinese chive increase the production of breast milk.

Preparation: Chinese chives are frequently added to soups, curries, and stir-fries. Leaves and flowers may be eaten raw or added to salads.

Topical Application: Chinese chive seeds are used to kill insects which have entered into the ear canal.

Preparation: As you roast seeds, allow the smoke to pass into the ear canal.

Chiretta, Chirata
Andrographis paniculata
Fa Thalaai

Action: Alterative, Antiallergic, Anti-inflammatory, Antipyretic, Astringent, Bitter Tonic, Blood Tonic, Cholagogue, Hepatic, Stomachic

Taste: Bitter   **Part Used:** Leaf, Bud, Young Shoot

Internal Application: Chiretta tea is reputed to be excellent for ailments of the upper respiratory system, including cold with congestion, sore throat, bronchitis, tonsillitis, hay fever, and other allergies. As a bitter tonic, it is particularly stimulating for the liver and increases production of bile. It has a beneficial effect on all liver and gall bladder disorders, as well as diabetes and hypoglycemia. Chiretta is a detoxifying herb, useful in cases of intestinal infection such as dysentery and other diarrhea, and in cleansing the blood. Chiretta is also used to relieve constipation, treat fever, and to reduce blood pressure.

Preparation: Tea from 1–5 handfuls fresh herb. Drink 3–4 times daily. Or powder dried herb; take 1.5 grams 3–4 times daily.

Topical Application: Fresh chiretta stalks are used to treat toothaches and abscesses.

Preparation: Chew raw stalks. Or pound leaves with mortar and pestle; mix with a bit of water; apply to affected area.

Caution: In larger doses, chiretta may cause nausea.

Note: *A. paniculata* is a local species of chiretta. Where it is not available, *Swertia chirata* (common chiretta) may be substituted.

Chrysanthemum
Chrysanthemum indicum
Geh Huay

Action: Alterative, Antipyretic, Antispasmodic, Bitter Tonic, Cardiac, Carminative, Diaphoretic, Emmenagogue, Hepatic, Nervine, Sedative, Stimulant

Taste: Bitter   **Part Used:** Flower

Internal Application: Iced chrysanthemum tea is one of the most popular drinks in Thailand, available at any market or restaurant. It is reputed to be a stimulant and tonic for the eyes, liver, heart, and nervous system. Therapeutically, chrysanthemum is used to treat all disorders of the liver and eyes, irregular or blocked menstruation, menstrual cramps, and PMS. It is also said to cure headaches and sore throat, to lower fever, and to calm the mind. It is a mildly bitter tonic, which can be sweetened with any natural sweetener to make a delicious hot or iced beverage.

Preparation: Drink tea 1–3 times daily, hot or iced.

Cinchona, Quinine Bark, Peruvian Bark
Cinchona officinalis, Cinchona succirubra

Action: Analgesic, Antipyretic, Antiseptic, Astringent, Bitter Tonic, Nervine, Stomachic

Taste: Bitter   **Part Used:** Bark

Internal Application: Until the advent of more potent synthetic medications, cinchona was the remedy of choice for malaria. It is still used for this purpose in isolated areas of rural Thailand and throughout South Asia in places where modern drugs and medical attention are unavailable. In smaller doses, cinchona is also useful for cases of influenza and fever, and as a daily bitter tonic to promote health and longevity.

Preparation: Tea. Drink 1–3 times daily.

Caution: In large doses, cinchona may cause headaches, dizziness, or stomach irritation. Cinchona may cause uterine contractions and should be avoided by pregnant women.

Cinnamon
Cinnamomum zeylanicum
Ob Chuey

Action: Alterative, Analgesic, Antiemetic, Antiseptic, Astringent, Cardiac, Carminative, Diaphoretic, Diuretic, Expectorant, Stimulant, Stomachic

Taste: Hot   **Part Used:** Bark, Leaf

Internal Application: Cinnamon is a stimulant for the kidneys, heart, and circulation, and is especially good in cases of chronic circulatory deficiency, hypotension, and chronic coldness. As a hot herb, cinnamon is used internally as a decongestant for colds and as a digestive against indigestion and sluggish digestion. The tea also counters nausea and vomiting, soothes constipation and gastrointestinal cramping, and promotes regular menstruation.

Preparation: Tea is made from dried cinnamon bark.

Topical Application: Cinnamon bark and leaf is used topically to soothe muscle aches and strains, as well as on the thoracic area to break up colds and congestion. This herb is also a topical analgesic and antiseptic useful for toothaches and mouth sores.

Preparation: Gargle with cinnamon tea, or apply directly to skin. Diluted in olive oil or other base oil, essential cinnamon oil can be applied directly to the skin on affected areas. (See *Homemade Tiger Balm™* in *Special Medicinal Recipes, Chapter V.*) Cinnamon leaves may also be used for this purpose and are one of the main ingredients in the traditional herbal sauna and compress (see *Chapter IV*).

Citronella Grass
Cymbopogon nardus, Cymbopogon winterianus
Ta Khrai Nom

Action: Blood Tonic, Carminative, Diaphoretic, Emmenagogue, Stimulant, Stomachic

Taste: Hot   **Part Used:** Leaf, Essential Oil, Rhizome

Internal Application: Infusion of citronella leaves is soothing to the stomach and helps counter flatulence, stomachache, indigestion, intestinal cramps, irritable bowel, and gastritis. The essential oil is also diaphoretic and stimulant, and promotes internal detoxification through encouraging sweating. The rhizome encourages regular menstruation, treats blocked menstruation, and halts excessive vaginal discharge. Citronella is used to induce labor, as it promotes uterine contractions. It also acts as a diuretic.

Preparation: Infusion of leaves or essential oil, decoction of rhizome.

Topical Application: Citronella is a natural insect repellent, and rural Thais place a bowl of pounded citronella leaves under the bed to ward off mosquitoes during the night. Decoction or infusion may also be applied to skin directly as insect repellent. Essential oil may be diluted in water and applied similarly.

Preparation: For insect repellent, apply citronella oil to a diffuser, or to a handkerchief placed over a light bulb. Citronella may be applied to the skin as well. Use 7% essential oil of citronella in 93% alcohol, or see *Herbs in Cosmetics* section in *Chapter III* for recipe.

Caution: Citronella should never be used internally by pregnant women.

Clove
Syzygium aromaticum
Kan Pluu

Action: Analgesic, Antiemetic, Antiseptic, Aphrodisiac, Blood Tonic, Carminative, Diaphoretic, Emmenagogue, Expectorant, Female Tonic, Lymphatic, Stimulant, Stomachic

Taste: Hot   **Part Used:** Flower

Internal Application: Like most hot herbs, clove is a digestion stimulant used traditionally to counter flatulence and indigestion. Hot herbs are also effective expectorants and are called for in cases of the common cold, especially with accompanying congestion. Clove is used frequently for this purpose, as well as for cough, bronchitis, lymph problems, and asthma. Clove tea is very effective for controlling nausea and vomiting, and is also used traditionally for lymph disease and uterine disorders. Due to its stimulating effect on the Fire element, clove tea warms the body, combating chronic coldness, hypothermia, chilblains, and frost-nip. The herb is reputed to have aphrodisiac qualities, although this is probably due to a general stimulating effect.

Preparation: Make tea from 3–4 crushed cloves in 1 cup (250 ml) boiling water. See also *Tea-Less Chai* recipe in *Chapter V.*

Topical Application: Topically, cloves have an antiseptic and analgesic effect, and they are therefore used both on the skin and in the mouth for sores and cuts. A gargle of tea is also beneficial for sore throat and toothaches.

Preparation: Make tea from 3–4 crushed cloves in 1 cup (250 ml) boiling water; apply topically when lukewarm with towel. (See also, *Homemade Tiger Balm*™ in *Chapter V.*)

Note: *S. aromaticum* is a locally occurring clove. Where it is not available, *Eugenia caryophyllata* (common clove) may be substituted.

Coconut
Cocos nucifera
Ma Phrao

Action: Diuretic, Emollient, Nutritive Tonic, Refrigerant

Taste: Sweet   **Part Used:** Meat of the coconut

Internal Application: The coconut palm is one of the most useful plants in Thailand. The fibrous husks of the coconut are used to make rope, mats, and brushes. Young green coconuts are prized for their sweet water, while the mature nut is shredded, mixed with hot water, and strained to produce coconut cream. An essential ingredient in Thai curries, coconut cream is frequently eaten as a nutritive tonic in cases of low immunity, low energy, emaciation, and wasting, and coconut milk may be used as a milk substitute for vegans or the lactose intolerant (although not as a replacement for infant formula).

Preparation: To make homemade coconut cream, grate one fresh coconut with a coconut shaver, fish-scaler, or other scraping instrument. Place grated coconut in a pan and cover with boiled water. Let stand until lukewarm. Strain coconut shavings with cheesecloth and set aside. Refrigerate liquid until cream separates. The thick cream will rise to the top of the container where it can be easily scraped off, leaving coconut milk underneath. (Dried grated coconut may be used to extract coconut milk, but will yield very little cream.)

Topical Application: Coconut oil is an indispensable ingredient in cosmetics, as well as cooking (see *Chapter III* for more information). As it possesses emollient properties, it is applied topically to burns, wounds, and skin lesions, to soothe pain and promote healing.

Preparation: Slowly mix together 1 part coconut oil with 1 part quicklime. Apply to skin.

Combretum
Combretum quadrangulare
Sa-kae

Action: Analgesic, Anthelmintic

Taste: Toxic   **Part Used:** Seed, Root, Leaf

Internal Application: Combretum seeds are used traditionally to purge tapeworms and other intestinal parasites. Decoction of the root is used to treat venereal disease, and decoction of the leaves is used to combat narcotic addiction. A poultice from the leaves is used topically to relieve muscular pain. The Wat Po texts further recommend combretum for treatment of bladder stones and abdominal distention.

Preparation: For anthelmintic, grind seeds finely to make powder. Take 1 tsp powder mixed with fried eggs. For other uses, make decoction from fresh or dried plant.

Corkwood Tree, Sesban
Sesbania grandiflora
Khae

Action: Antipyretic, Astringent, Hemostatic

Taste: Astringent **Part Used:** Leaf, Stem-bark

Internal Application: The bark of the corkwood tree stem is an astringent used to combat diarrhea and dysentery. The fresh leaves are used to treat fever.

Preparation: Decoction from fire-roasted bark or leaves. Fresh flowers, shoots, and young leaves may be steamed and eaten with chili sauce.

Topical Application: Decoction of the stem-bark is used topically on wounds and cuts as a hemostatic.

Crocodile
Jarakae

Action: Bitter Tonic, Blood Tonic, Female Tonic

Taste: Bitter **Part Used:** Bile from gall-bladder of Crocodylus siamensis

Internal Application: Crocodile bile is an expensive but sought-after tonic for the uterus and other female reproductive organs, used immediately following pregnancy. It is traditionally held to be a bitter tonic for longevity and the blood in both sexes and to treat low immunity, low energy, fainting, and vertigo.

Culantro
Eryngium foetidum
Phak-chee farang

Action: Blood Tonic, Laxative, Purgative **Part Used:** Leaf, Bud, Young Shoot

Internal Application: The Hill-Tribes use this herb to flavor soups and curries. Medicinally, it is used as a laxative and as a detoxifying purgative for malaria, allergic reactions, and poisonous insect bites. Another species, the Amethyst Holly (*E. amethystinum*) is also used for these purposes, as well as for increased immunity, chronic colds, and general longevity.

Preparation: Decoction

Cuttlefish
Pla Muuk

Action: Nutritive Tonic

Taste: Salty **Part Used:** Meat of Sepia opp.

Internal Application: Cuttlefish is considered a nutritive tonic which promotes general health and well-being. As a regular part of the diet, it is also said to be a remedy for chronic diseases of the teeth and gums, for mouth sores, acne, and skin diseases.

Preparation: Eat fish steamed or smoked.

Daeng
Xylia xylocarpa

Action: Antipyretic, Astringent, Female Tonic, Laxative, Pectoral, Tonic

Part Used: Whole plant

Internal Application: The flower of the daeng is a cardiac tonic and is also prescribed for fever. The stem-bark is traditionally used to counter fever as well, and is an antidiarrheal. Decoction of the wood is a laxative and is a tonic used to treat uterine, ovarian, and lung diseases and cancers. Either the wood or the stem-bark can be used daily as an astringent to counter internal bleeding and blood in the vomit, stool, or vaginal discharge.

Preparation: Take decoction once daily.

Damask Rose
Rosa damascena
Kulaap Mon

Action: Alterative, Astringent, Calmative, Carminative, Cholagogue, Emmenagogue, Laxative, Nervine, Refrigerant, Sedative

Taste: Aromatic   **Part Used:** Flower

Internal Application: Rosewater is a common ingredient in Asian desserts. Hot or cold, rose infusion may be used as a stimulant to counter low immunity, low energy, and chronic fatigue. The tea is a cholagogue, or bile stimulant, which aids in digestion and assimilation of nutrients, and encourages regular menstruation. Rose flowers are added to the traditional sauna or steam bath for eye disorders and infections, and for a relaxing effect on nervous disorders, anxiety, insomnia, tension headaches, and stress.

Preparation: Rosewater can be made by cold infusion of a large quantity of rose flowers in water. Let sit overnight. To make hot rose tea, heat rosewater to temperature without boiling. Ayurvedic herbalists macerate rose flowers in honey, and administer the remedy by the spoonful. This recipe is very soothing for sore throats. For more information on sauna and steam, see *Chapter IV.*

Note: Rose Otto essential oil may be substituted for Damask Rose, provided it is 100% pure.

Datura
Datura metel
Lanpong Khao

Action: Antiemetic, Antiparasitic, Antipyretic, Antiseptic, Antitussive, Expectorant, Nervine, Tonic

Taste: Toxic   **Part Used:** Whole plant

Internal Application: The Wat Po texts mention datura as a remedy for many ailments. Powder from the dried seeds of the datura plant is used in small doses to treat fever and as a cerebral tonic. The flower is dried and smoked by asthmatics as a bronchodilator and also curbs nausea. Decoction of the root is also used to treat asthma, as well as bronchitis and cough. Decoction of the leaves is used traditionally to treat mucous or blood in the stool, and the juice of the fruit is administered in drops to treat infections of the ear.

Topical Application: A poultice made from the seeds of the datura is used topically to treat ringworm and other skin parasites. This poultice, or a decoction from the fresh root, may be used to treat toothache and abscesses. A poultice from fresh flowers is applied to wounds, bruises, sprains, and sore muscles by some Hill-Tribes.

Preparation: Powder from dried seeds; mix with hot water to make paste. Apply to affected areas.

Caution: The old texts warn that small doses improve the memory, but overdose causes insanity. Always use datura with caution, as there are many varieties, some of which are extremely poisonous, and many of which are potent hallucinogens.

Ebony Tree
Diospyros mollis
Ma Kluea

Action: Anthelmintic, Tonic

Taste: Toxic (root, fruit); Salty (bark)   **Part Used:** Root, Fruit, Bark

Internal Application: The fruits of the ebony tree are used traditionally to make a black dye for cloth. Medicinally, they are used to purge the intestines of tapeworms and other parasites. The Wat Po texts mention ebony tree root as a remedy for vomiting and nausea, and the bark as a remedy for emaciation or wasting associated with chronic illnesses.

Preparation: Adult dosage is 25 fruits. For children 10 years and over, the dosage is 1 fruit per year of age, up to maximum of 25. Mash raw fresh fruit with mortar and pestle. Soak in coconut milk. Strain and drink before breakfast.

Caution: Not for use by children under 10 years of age, post-partum women, or anyone with gastrointestinal complaints. Use with caution, as overdose may cause blindness.

Emblic Myrobalan, Indian Gooseberry
Phyllanthus emblica, Emblica officinalis
Ma Khaam Bom

Action: Antioxidant, Antipyretic, Antitussive, Aphrodisiac, Astringent, Blood Tonic, Diuretic, Expectorant, Hemostatic, Hepatic, Laxative, Nutritive Tonic, Refrigerant, Stomachic

Taste: Sour   **Part Used:** Fruit

Internal Application: The emblic myrobalan is used traditionally for respiratory afflictions, including colds, congestion, cough, and asthma, as well as for indigestion. The fruit is one of the highest natural sources of vitamin C and is a traditional daily tonic for the brain, nervous system, blood, bones, liver, spleen, stomach, heart, eyes, hair, bones, nails, teeth, and gums. Because of its detoxifying and antioxidant properties, emblic myrobalan is especially beneficial for those with frequent colds, low immunity, smokers, and those who live in polluted environments. In Thailand, the dried, pickled fruits are sold in bags, and are eaten like we in the West would eat prunes. Emblic myrobalan is one of the most commonly used herbs in the Ayurvedic system, employed to increase immunity, regulate the digestive system, and to treat fever, internal bleeding, diabetes, hypoglycemia, gout, gastritis, hepatitis and other liver disease, jaundice, constipation, diarrhea, hemorrhoids, anxiety, stress, chronic fatigue, low immunity, low energy, osteoporosis, and for aiding in convalescence from chronic disease.

Preparation: Two to five raw fruits are mashed with mortar and pestle, salted, and sucked 3–4 times throughout the day. For daily consumption, jellied or pickled fruits are highly recommended. Emblic myrobalan may also be powdered or taken in decoction. Use 250 mg – 1000 mg.

Note: Thai healers may use *Phyllanthus urinaria*, called "Yaa Tai Bai," as a substitute.

Eucalyptus
Eucalyptus globulus, others

Action: Antiseptic, Antispasmodic, Antitussive, Expectorant, Diaphoretic, Nervine, Pectoral, Stimulant

Taste: Hot and Aromatic   **Part Used:** Leaf, Oil

Internal Application: Eucalyptus is a popular herbal remedy in Thailand, and it has even become somewhat fashionable among young Thais to carry around a vial of eucalyptus and peppermint oil for frequent sniffing. There are many species of eucalyptus, most of which can be used medicinally. Eucalyptus is an extremely effective treatment for colds, especially those with excessive congestion of the sinus and/or lungs, as well as cough, bronchitis, asthma, sore throat, and other respiratory ailments. Symptoms are relieved by inhalation of the vapors, by tea, or by topical application to chest, throat, and under the nose. Eucalyptus tea is also good for indigestion and fever. Hill-Tribes use eucalyptus tea internally as an analgesic and a cold remedy, and the inhalation to stop nosebleeds.

Preparation: Bruise leaves with mortar and pestle; add to sauna or steam bath, or apply to chest and back with hot herbal compress (see *Chapter IV*). Essential oil of eucalyptus may be used as a substitute in most cases, but only if pure. Tea can be made by infusing 2 fresh or 4 dried eucalyptus leaves.

Topical Application: The eucalyptus is one of the most potent antiseptic and antibacterial herbs. Leaves are used topically on ulcers, infections, and sores of the skin, and may be safely applied to burns. A poultice may also be used on sprains, bruises, and sore muscles. A few fresh leaves or a small amount of pure eucalyptus oil may be mixed with warm water and used as a gargle for sore throats, cough, and mouth sores.

Preparation: Mash leaves with mortar and pestle; mix with hot water. Apply directly to affected area. Essential oil of eucalyptus can be used as substitute in topical applications. Apply a small amount directly to the skin with a hot towel.

Caution: Taken internally in large doses, eucalyptus may be poisonous. Take care when using essential oils to adjust dosage.

False Daisy
Eclipta prostrate, Eclipta alba
Kameng

Action: Alterative, Antiparasitic, Antipyretic, Blood Tonic, Carminative, Hemostatic, Hepatic, Laxative, Tonic, Vulnerary

Taste: Bitter   **Part Used:** Whole plant

Internal Application: The whole plant of the false daisy is used to treat chest infections, asthma, and bronchitis. It is a carminative used to expel gas from the lower intestines. It is also considered to be a longevity tonic and a tonic for the liver, spleen, and blood, and it is used to treat cirrhosis, hepatitis, and anemia. The leaf and root are used as a laxative. The root is used for cases of flatulence, temporary paralysis, and fainting or feeling of exhaustion post-partum. The juice of the stem is prescribed for jaundice.

Preparation: Decoction

Topical Application: A poultice of the false daisy may be used topically for skin diseases and ringworm. The decoction may be added to olive or coconut oil and massaged into the scalp as a hair tonic to prevent hair loss and early greying. The same oil may also be used as a topical anti-inflammatory.

Finger Root
Boesenbergia pandurata, Boesenbergia rotunda
Krachai

Action: Anthelmintic, Antiallergic, Carminative, Digestive, Stomachic

Taste: Hot   **Part Used:** Root, Leaf

Internal Application: Finger root is a common ingredient in Thai soups and curries. As a digestive, it is traditionally included in the diet to aid sluggish digestion, flatulence, and indigestion. The rhizome is also used for tooth and gum disease, diarrhea, dysentery, and as a general diuretic. Tea made from the finger root leaves is employed in cases of food poisoning and allergic reactions to food.

Preparation: Mash fresh root with mortar and pestle, and make decoction. Or make powder from dried or fire-roasted root.

Foetid Cassia
Cassia tora
Nha lap meun

Action: Anthelmintic, Antipruritic, Antipyretic, Diuretic, Laxative, Purgative, Sedative

Taste: Bitter   **Part Used:** Seed, Stem, Root

Internal Application: Decoction of foetid cassia seeds is preferred in cases of acute constipation and intestinal worms for its purging action on the bowels. It is also used to calm fevers, to lessen inflammation of the eyes, to lower high blood pressure and cholesterol, as a diuretic, and as a sedative. Decoction of the stem and/or root is also diuretic and may be used topically to stop itching.

Preparation: Roast dried seeds in pan. Make decoction by boiling seeds in 1 pint (500 ml) water. Use 10–13 g seeds for laxative; 5–10 g for diuretic. Fresh leaves may be boiled or steamed, and eaten with chili sauce for milder effect.

Galangal, Ginza, Siamese Ginger
Alpinia galanga, Alpinia officinarum, Alpinia nigra
Khaa

Action: Antiemetic, Antiparasitic, Antiseptic, Aphrodisiac, Carminative, Diaphoretic, Digestive, Expectorant, Stimulant, Stomachic, Tonic

Taste: Hot   **Part Used:** Rhizome

Internal Application: Galangal is used in Thai medicine in a very similar way to ginger. Ginger is considered to be a superior herb, but galangal is more common in Thailand. Its flavor is distinctive, and galangal is an indispensable ingredient in Thai soups and curries. It is the key ingredient in the Thai national dish, *Tom Yam* soup (see *Chapter III* for recipe). As a hot herb, the galangal rhizome has a stimulating effect on the digestion, and is therefore useful in cases of indigestion, flatulence, and stomachache. It is also recommended for diarrhea, nausea, and seasickness. Galangal is reputed to be an aphrodisiac, although this is probably due to its general stimulating effect on the Fire element.

Preparation: Decoction from one "thumb-length" (or about 5 grams) fresh galangal, finely chopped, grated, or mashed with mortar and pestle. Boil 10–15 minutes; drink after meals.

Topical Application: Galangal has an antiseptic action similar to ginger and may be used topically for bacterial and fungal skin infections, acne, mosquito bites, bee stings, other insect bites, and as a gargle for mouth sores. *A. nigra* is used for treatment of ringworm and other skin parasites.

Preparation: Mash fresh galangal with mortar and pestle. Add a bit of water to make a paste; apply topically to skin. For treatment of skin parasites, add 1 part galangal to 3 parts alcohol and let sit overnight before applying. For sores within the mouth, gargle with galangal tea.

Gandaria, Plum Mango
Bouea macrophylla
Maprang

Action: Antipyretic, Blood Tonic, Expectorant, Laxative

Taste: Sour   **Part Used:** Fruit

Internal Application: Gandaria is a small fruit with flavor similar to a mango but with the appearance of a plum. It is used traditionally as a treatment for fever, congestion of the bronchi, mouth sores, and constipation. It is also used to detoxify the blood.

Preparation: Eat raw fruit.

Garden Balsam, Impatiens
Impatiens balsamica
Thian baan

Action: Antipruritic, Tonic   **Part Used:** Leaf

Topical Application: Garden balsam leaves are applied topically to eczema, skin ulcers, insect bites, allergic reactions, hives, sores, wounds, and bacterial infection of the skin and nails. The Hill-Tribes use the garden balsam topically for inflammation and low immunity, and internally as a general tonic and as an aid in the delivery of babies.

Preparation: Pound leaves with mortar and pestle. Apply to affected areas 3 times daily.

Garcinia
Garcinia indica, Garcinia cambogia
Som kak

Action: Alterative, Anthelmintic, Antitumor, Digestive

Part Used: Fruit

Internal Application: Garcinia aids in weight loss by accelerating the metabolism of fats and carbohydrates. It is safe for long-term use and has been the subject of numerous tests in the U.S. and Europe as a natural alternative to chemical weight-loss drugs. It is used in Thailand as a dietary supplement for suppressing the appetite. It is also used traditionally for constipation, edema, intestinal parasites, sluggish digestion, and for increasing body heat. It is being researched for antitumor and anticancerous properties.

Preparation: Decoction from dried fruit, or grind dried fruit to make powder.

Garlic
Allium sativum
Krathiam

Action: Alterative, Anthelmintic, Antipyretic, Antirheumatic, Antiseptic, Antispasmodic, Antitussive, Aphrodisiac, Blood Tonic, Cardiac, Carminative, Cholagogue, Digestive, Diuretic, Expectorant, Hepatic, Refrigerant, Stimulant, Stomachic, Tonic

Taste: Hot   **Part Used:** Bulb

Internal Application: Along with ginger, garlic is one of the most useful herbs in Eastern and Western traditions alike. Garlic is one of the most commonly used herbs in Thai cuisine and is a key ingredient in many Thai dishes. (See *Chapter III* for some recipe ideas.) As with most hot herbs, garlic is a digestive with carminative action of particular use in cases of flatulence and indigestion. Hot herbs are also effective expectorants successfully used to fight colds, congestion, asthma, bronchitis, and cough. Garlic is a potent detoxifying agent and is therefore beneficial in fighting liver disease, toxic colon, and in general detoxification of the blood and organs. In large doses, garlic has a purgative effect on intestinal worms and other parasites, and is used to prevent malaria and dengue (it is said that mosquitoes won't bite one who eats garlic frequently). Other diseases benefited by garlic include arthritis, heart disease, gall bladder disease, fever, and cystitis. Garlic reputedly lowers blood cholesterol, lowers high blood pressure, raises low blood pressure, and is recognized in many cultures the world over as a stimulating aphrodisiac.

Preparation: Eat 2–4 cloves daily raw or cooked in food.

Topical Application: As a powerful antiseptic, garlic may be applied topically to bacterial and fungal skin infections, superficial wounds, dermatitis, and swelling. A few drops of garlic juice in the ears fights ear infections, and in the nose, fights sinusitis. Rubbing the temples with garlic cloves is a classic remedy for relieving headache.

Preparation: Mash raw cloves with mortar and pestle; mix with warm water to make a paste, and apply directly to affected areas.

Ginger
Zingiber officinale
Khing

Action: Adjuvant, Analgesic, Antiemetic, Anti-inflammatory, Antirheumatic, Antiseptic, Antitussive, Aphrodisiac, Carminative, Diaphoretic, Digestive, Emmenagogue, Expectorant, Galactogogue, Stimulant, Stomachic, Tonic

Taste: Hot **Part Used:** Rhizome

Internal Application: Ginger is the quintessential panacea in the Thai herbal pharmacopoeia. As a hot herb, ginger is a powerful stimulant, especially of the digestive tract. It is the herb of choice for stimulation of digestion, and is used to combat flatulence, indigestion, gastritis, peptic ulcer, diarrhea, sluggish digestion, nausea, and vomiting. Ginger tea is also used for colds, congestion, sore throat, fevers, nausea, seasickness, mouth sores, insomnia, heart disease, arthritis, irregular or blocked menstruation, chronic back pain, hemorrhoids, and beri-beri (vitamin B1 deficiency), earning it the reputation as a cure-all. Hill-Tribe healers give ginger tea to mothers immediately following birth to promote health and rapid recovery. Ginger also acts as a galactagogue, encouraging production of breast milk. Ginger is used as an adjuvant in many herbal preparations in order to lessen side effects and increase the potency of other herbs, and is the most frequently used herb in this collection.

Preparation: Decoction from one "thumb-length" (or about 5 grams) fresh ginger, finely chopped, grated, or mashed with mortar and pestle. Boil 10–15 minutes; drink after meals. For cough and cold, add lemon juice. (See also *Zingiber Tea* in *Special Medicinal Recipes, Chapter V.*)

Topical Application: Ginger has a powerful antiseptic action and may be used topically for bacterial and fungal skin infections, parasites, and acne.

Preparation: Mash fresh ginger with mortar and pestle. Add a bit of alcohol to make a paste; apply topically to skin. For sores within the mouth, gargle with ginger tea and a pinch of salt. (See also *Herbs in Cosmetics* in *Chapter III* for skin-care recipes using ginger and *Chapter IV* for herbal compress recipes.)

Gingko
Gingko biloba
Gingko

Action: Antioxidant, Antitussive, Astringent, Expectorant, Nervine, Stimulant

Part Used: Leaf

Internal Application: Gingko improves blood circulation, particularly to the brain, and is commonly prescribed to older individuals to maintain mental acuity through old age and to counter or prevent Alzheimer's disease and other memory loss. It may also be used by younger individuals to enhance memory and mental clarity, and as a rich source of detoxifying antioxidants. Gingko has also been shown to have a beneficial effect on depression, mood swings, arthritis, arteriosclerosis, stress, anxiety, bronchitis, and can be used to treat varicose veins and other disorders due to chronic circulatory deficiency.

Preparation: Gingko tea should be taken 2–3 times daily for 3 months for noticeable effect. It is often mixed with Gotu Kola in a 1 to 1 ratio.

Ginseng
Panax ginseng
Soam

Action: Alterative, Antiallergic, Antiemetic, Aphrodisiac, Blood Tonic, Cardiac, Demulcent, Male Tonic, Nervine, Nutritive Tonic, Stimulant, Stomachic, Tonic

Taste: Hot and Sweet **Part Used:** Rhizome

Internal Application: Ginseng is an example of an herb prized by Chinese medicine that has made its way into the Thai tradition. Almost every sizable grocery store in Thailand has a well-stocked shelf of ginseng extracts and products imported from China or Korea. The extract of the ginseng rhizome is said to be the best longevity tonic for males and is frequently taken by men over 50 on a daily basis. It is held to be a powerful aphrodisiac and a sure cure for impotence, premature ejaculation, and other male sexual dysfunctions. For both sexes, it is a cardiac tonic which helps strengthen the heart and circulatory system, while reducing cholesterol and controlling blood sugar. Ginseng is used as a stimulant for the entire system and to counter low immunity, low energy, chronic fatigue, stress, debility, and emaciation. As a demulcent, ginseng is also useful in cases of nausea, vomiting, sinusitis, hay fever, and other allergies. It is also used to treat blood diseases, irregular menstruation, colds, and bronchial infections.

Preparation: Ginseng extract is the most commonly available form of this herb, although the fresh rhizome is used in some tonic food recipes and decoction can be made with the root. Extract should be taken before breakfast, and should not be taken with caffeine. Dosage differs according to strength of extract, but the average dose is 2–10 ml. Ginger may be used as an adjuvant for heightened stimulating effect. (See *Zingiber Tea* in *Special Medicinal Recipes, Chapter V.*)

Golden Shower, Purging Cassia
Cassia fistula
Khuun

Action: Antipyretic, Expectorant, Laxative, Purgative, Stimulant, Tonic

Taste: Astringent   **Part Used:** Seed Pod, Flower

Internal Application: The black, sticky pulp surrounding the seeds of the golden shower is used traditionally as a laxative and expectorant. In larger doses, it is a purgative. Tea from the flower is also a laxative and an antipyretic. Hill-Tribes use the flowers in the steam bath or sauna to treat vertigo, low energy, and fainting, and as a general tonic for health and longevity.

Preparation: Boil 4 g of the pulp of the seed pod with salt. Strain; drink at bedtime. Alternatively, boil seeds in water with salt until soft; eat seeds at bedtime. For more information on steam bath and sauna, see *Chapter IV.*

Gotu Kola, Brahmi, Asiatic Pennywort
Centella asiatica (synonym: Hydrocotyle asiatica)
Bua Bok

Action: Alterative, Antioxidant, Antipyretic, Antirheumatic, Astringent, Bitter Tonic, Blood Tonic, Diuretic, Emmolient, Expectorant, Hepatic, Nervine, Vulnerary

Taste: Bitter   **Part Used:** Leaf, Stem

Internal Application: Gotu kola is primarily a tonic for the nervous system, promoting clarity of thinking, mental calmness, and emotional balance. It is used to treat psychological disorders, chemical imbalances of the brain, memory loss, Alzheimer's, and epilepsy. It is high in vitamin A and is considered to be an excellent daily tonic for old age. It has an especially beneficial effect on the immune system, veins, liver, spleen, and gall bladder. As a blood purifier, it is also used to counter colds, fever, arthritis, all types of skin diseases, urinary tract infections, sexually transmitted diseases, hepatitis, and uterine cancer. Tea made from the fresh leaf is used to treat sore throat, fevers, and diarrhea.

Preparation: Drink tea made from dried leaves and stem once daily for 1 month. Use honey as an adjuvant. Or extract juice from fresh leaves, dilute, and bring to a boil. Sweeten with honey before drinking. Gotu kola is often taken with Gingko (see previous page).

Topical Application: Gotu kola is applied topically to soothe burns and to help in healing wounds. The leaf has antifungal and antibacterial properties, and is used to treat staphylococcus infections.

Preparation: Mash a handful of leaves with mortar and pestle, adding just enough water to make a paste. Apply to affected areas as needed.

Caution: Excessive doses of gotu kola may cause nausea and/or vomiting.

Green Tea
Camellia sinensis
Cha-keay

Action: Anti-inflammatory, Antioxidant, Astringent, Bitter Tonic, Cardiac, Digestive, Diuretic, Stomachic

Taste: Bitter   **Part Used:** Leaf

Internal Application: Green tea is possibly the most popular beverage in Asia, although Thailand's consumption is somewhat less than China's or Japan's. Mostly, green tea's beneficial properties are due to tannins, antibiotic alkaloids that occur naturally in the leaf. In modern times, green tea has been shown to be rich in antioxidants, which seems to confirm its long-standing reputation as a general tonic. Taken regularly, green tea promotes a healthy immune system, protecting against infections and cancers of the respiratory and digestive systems. Green tea has a regulating and alkalizing effect on the digestive system and helps both constipation and diarrhea. In general it is useful as a digestive, although different processing and roasting methods produce differing results. Green tea also is beneficial for blood circulation, aids in disinfecting bacterial infections of the mouth, and protects against tooth and gum disease.

Preparation: Tea

Topical Application: Applied topically, green tea is an anti-inflammatory for burns and skin irritations.

Preparation: Soak leaves in hot water; apply lukewarm leaves to affected areas.

Note: Black tea is made from the oxidized leaves of *C. sinensis* but does not share all of green tea's therapeutic qualities.

Guava
Psidium guajava
Farang

Action: Antiseptic, Astringent, Emmenagogue, Laxative, Sedative

Taste: Astringent   **Part Used:** Leaf, Fruit

Internal Application: Guava is most commonly prescribed traditionally for diarrhea because of the astringent qualities of the leaves and unripe fruit. It is also useful to treat cases of blocked or irregular menstruation, and cases of chronic stress or anxiety.

Preparation: Flame-roast 10–15 leaves until yellow in color. Boil in 1 pint (500 ml) water. Take 1/2 cup (125 ml) decoction every 3 hours as needed. Powder may also be made from the unripe fruit by removing the seeds, drying, and grinding. Take 1 tsp dry or in hot water. For a gentler effect, the unripe fruit may also be eaten fresh, dipped into a mixture of sugar, salt, and chili powder. Or unripe guava may be juiced and drunk with a pinch of salt.

Schefflera leucantha, Schefflera venulosa
Hanuman Prasan Kai

Action: Antitussive, Astringent, Hemostatic

Taste: Astringent   **Part Used:** Fresh Leaf

Internal Application: The leaf of this plant is astringent and drying, and is used to treat colds, respiratory tract infections, cough, asthma, and difficulty breathing. It is also employed in cases of cough; blood in the vomit, stool, or vaginal discharge; and internal bleeding for its hemostatic effect.

Preparation: Decoction from 7–8 clusters of leaves. Take twice daily, before breakfast and dinner.

Topical Application: Poultice may be applied topically as a hemostatic to contusions, cuts, and bleeding wounds.

Preparation: Apply topically with poultice or cold compress.

Heart-Leaved Moonseed
Tinospora tuberculata, Tinospora crispa
Boraphet

Action: Antipyretic, Appetizer, Bitter Tonic, Lymphatic, Pectoral, Stomachic

Taste: Bitter   **Part Used:** Stem

Internal Application: Boraphet (pronounced "bora-pet") is used to treat any disease in which fever is the initial symptom. It also stimulates the appetite and is considered to be a bitter tonic especially beneficial for the lungs, bile, and lymphatic system. The Wat Po texts mention boraphet as a cure for intestinal parasites, stomach problems in babies, malaria, eye and ear disease, and for mucous congestion.

Preparation: A foot-long segment of stem (about 30–40 grams) is pounded with a mortar and pestle. Mashed stalks are soaked in water, and strained. Decoction is drunk twice daily until fever is gone. Or one inch of fresh stem is chewed with lots of water 2–3 times daily.

Note: *T. baenzigeri,* may also be used.

Henna
Lawsonia inermis
Thian King

Action: Alterative, Antiparasitic, Antipyretic, Antiseptic

Taste: Bitter   **Part Used:** Leaf

Topical Application: Powdered henna leaf is widely used in India to dye hair. The fresh leaf may be applied as a topical antiseptic to fungal and/or bacterial infections of the skin and nails. It is also used to treat ringworm and may be used orally as a gargle for mouth and gum disease or infections.

Preparation: Mash fresh leaf with mortar and pestle, mixing with equal quantity of turmeric and a pinch of salt. Make poultice.

Hibiscus, Roselle
Hibiscus sabdariffa
Krachiap Daeng

Action: Antitussive, Carminative, Diuretic, Expectorant, Refrigerant, Tonic

Taste: Astringent **Part Used:** Flower, Seed

Internal Application: Hibiscus tea or juice is primarily prescribed as a diuretic for cases of gallstones, kidney stones, and urinary tract infections. It is additionally used to treat indigestion, flatulence, peptic ulcer, fever, cough, hypertension, kidney cramps, and back pain. It is high in calcium and therefore is added to the daily diet to treat and prevent tooth and bone deterioration. Hibiscus flower is held to lower blood cholesterol. The seed is also a diuretic, and is a tonic for the four elements.

Preparation: Tea from dried flowers. Drink 3 times daily. Or take 3 g seed daily in powdered form.

Holy Basil, Sacred Basil
Ocymum sanctum
Kaphrao Daeng

Action: Antipyretic, Antirheumatic, Antispasmodic, Antitussive, Carminative, Diaphoretic, Laxative, Nervine, Stomachic

Taste: Hot **Part Used:** Whole plant

Internal Application: Holy basil is so called because it is considered sacred in many parts of South Asia. In India, where it is the favored herbs of the Brahmins, it is said to promote spiritual purity and to strengthen the mind. While not necessarily considered sacred in Thailand, this herb is indispensable in cooking and is the primary condiment for most Thai soups and curries. (See *Chapter III* for some recipe ideas.)

Holy basil is a common ingredient in treatments for colds and flu. It is the perfect digestive and is a simple remedy for gastritis, irritable bowel, indigestion, flatulence, nausea, and vomiting. As an antispasmodic, it is useful for any stomach or intestinal cramping, including those caused by irritable bowel syndrome, peptic ulcer, gastritis, and pre-menstrual syndrome. Holy basil is also used in treatments for easing headaches, cough, sinusitis, and arthritis. While the herb may be used to combat constipation, the seeds are more effective laxatives. Some Hill-Tribes use basil in the steam bath or sauna for eye infections or pain, and topically as a poultice for fungal infections.

Preparation: Make tea from fresh leaves, flowers, and stalks. Take after meals as a digestive aid. For laxative, soak 2 tsps seeds in water for several hours. Seeds should take up a full glass when fully bloated. Take before bed. See *Chapter IV* for steam-bath and sauna.

Note: Where *O. sanctum* is unavailable, *O. basilicum,* or common basil, may be substituted.

Honey
Nam Pueng

Action: Adjuvant, Antitussive, Demulcent, Emollient, Nutritive Tonic

Taste: Sweet   **Part Used:** Raw, unprocessed Honey

Internal Application: Honey has a soothing effect on the throat and is typically used in traditional Thai herbalism as an adjuvant, or helping herb, with other remedies, especially treatments of colds, cough, sore throat, and asthma. Raw honey contributes to general strength and well-being, and is therefore used in nutritive preparations for longevity and convalescence, as well as in general tonics. In the case of cough and sore throat, it may be taken by the spoonful as necessary to soothe symptoms.

Preparation: Honey is typically administered with powders or dried herbs, or as a sweetener in herbal tea. (See *Special Medicinal Recipes, Chapter V,* for cold remedies.)

Horseradish Tree, Moringo
Moringa oleifera
Mahum

Action: Antirheumatic, Antiseptic, Astringent, Carminative, Digestive, Hemostatic, Stomachic, Vulnerary

Taset: Hot   **Part Used:** Bark, Root, Seed

Internal Application: Decoction of the bark of the horseradish tree is a digestion stimulant used traditionally for combating flatulence, indigestion, and bloated stomach.

Preparation: Decoction. The young shoots and flowers may alternatively be steamed and eaten with chili sauce or in soups.

Topical Application: Decoction of the root is a disinfectant and may be used as an astringent to stop bleeding and help promote the healing of wounds. The seeds, when roasted and ground, are made into a poultice for arthritis.

Indian Marsh Fleabane
Pluchea indica
Khlu

Action: Diuretic, Tonic   **Part Used:** Leaf

Internal Application: Indian marsh fleabane is considered to be an excellent longevity tonic. It is used therapeutically for its diuretic action, especially for cases of hemorrhoids, diabetes, and hypoglycemia.

Preparation: Flame-roast 15–20 leaves until yellow. Make decoction. Drink 3 times daily before meals.

Ironweed
Vernonia cinerea
Seua Saam Khaa

Action: Antirheumatic, Antitussive, Bitter Tonic, Digestive, Emmenagogue, Stomachic

Taste: Bitter   **Part Used:** Leaf, Flower, Rhizome

Internal Application: Ironweed is a Thai cure-all and is often used as a detoxifying bitter tonic for daily consumption. It is prescribed in cases of diabetes and hypoglycemia to help control blood sugar and to prevent sores and skin ulcers. It is successfully used as well for colds and respiratory disorders such as cough and asthma, arthritis, urinary tract infections, blocked or irregular menstruation, jaundice, back pain, and beri-beri (or vitamin B1 deficiency). Thais trying to quit smoking drink ironweed tea daily to help overcome the side effects associated with nicotine withdrawal. Ironweed is also a digestive which promotes the natural processes of the digestive system, offering relief from stomachaches and peptic ulcers.

Preparation: Make tea with 1 tsp rhizome or with equivalent amount of leaves and/or flowers. Drink 2 times daily, before meals.

Ironwood
Mesua ferrea
Boun Nark

Action: Antipyretic, Astringent, Blood Tonic, Cardiac, Stimulant, Tonic, Vulnerary

Taste: Aromatic   **Part Used:** Flower

Internal Application: Tea made from the dried ironwood flower is an astringent used traditionally as a tonic for the four elements. It has a beneficial effect on the blood and heart, and is used in cases of low energy, chronic fatigue, low immunity, hypertension, and fever. Ironwood may also be used in the steam bath or sauna, and the vapor is especially beneficial to the eyes.

Preparation: Make tea from dried flowers, or add to sauna or steam bath. (See *Chapter IV*).

Ivy Gourd
Coccinia indica, Coccinia grandis
Tam Loeng

Action: Antipruritic, Antipyretic, Purgative, Tonic

Taste: Bland   **Part Used:** Leaf

Internal Application: Ivy gourd leaves are taken in decoction as a purgative and as a detoxifier for food poisoning. It lowers fevers and is used by some Hill-Tribes as a tonic for general health and strength.

Preparation: Decoction.

Topical Application: Ivy gourd is applied topically to insect bites, hives, allergic rashes, itching, inflamed wounds, and rashes from poisonous plants.

Preparation: Mash leaves with mortar and pestle. Mix with alumina clay and a bit of water to make a paste. Apply to affected area.

Jackfruit
Artocarpus integrifolia, Artocarpus heterophyllus
Kanoon

Action: Demulcent, Nutritive Tonic

Taste: Oily   **Part Used:** Seed, Root

Internal Application: The jackfruit is an enormous fruit which often grows up to 3 feet in length. The heartwood of the jackfruit tree is used by monks in rural Northeastern Thailand's Forest Tradition monasteries to dye their robes. Chips of wood are boiled in water, producing a rich earth-tone dye called "gaen-kanun," which is held to have remarkable medicinal qualities. In fact, monks of this tradition never wash their robes. Once a week, the robes are re-boiled in jackfruit dye, and are hung to dry in the sun. Robes treated in this manner are said to never smell bad, and monks swear by the protection the dyed robes impart to the skin—such as immunity from fungal infections, skin disorders, and disagreeable body odor.

All over Thailand, the fleshy tulip-shaped segments of the jackfruit are eaten raw when ripe and are cooked in curries when unripe. The seed is a tonic for promotion of general health and invigoration of energy. The seeds are boiled or roasted, and are eaten in curry. As it is a nutritive tonic high in caloric energy, jackfruit seed is especially useful in convalescence, in cases of low immunity, low energy, chronic fatigue, or chronic illness, and in old age. Decoction of the root is used to treat diarrhea.

Jasmine
Jasminum officinale
Mali

Action: Alterative, Antipyretic, Antiseptic, Astringent, Cardiac, Emmenagogue, Nervine, Sedative

Taste: Aromatic   **Part Used:** Flower

Internal Application: Jasmine flowers are considered by Buddhists to be sacred, and they play a part in any temple ceremony in Thailand. Strung into garlands, they are often hung from the rear-view mirrors of cars as a talisman against misfortune and are placed by devotees at the foot of Buddha statues as an offering.

Jasmine flowers are common ingredients in the herbal steam baths or saunas. The Wat Po texts prescribe many different species of jasmine for snake bite, smallpox, diarrhea, dysentery, chest pain, fever, convulsions, poisoning, and tetanus. The vapor of *Jasminum officinale* is a calmative for stress, anxiety, nervousness, and panic attacks. Jasmine inhalations and tea are both beneficial for disorders, diseases, and infections of the eyes, as well as for heart disease, fever, and chronic thirst. Jasmine is being researched for its anticancerous properties.

Preparation: Tea may be made with fresh or dried flowers. For steam-bath and sauna preparations, see *Chapter IV.*

Note: There are many species of jasmine that may be used medicinally. See also Arabian Jasmine and Night Jasmine in this collection.

Jewel Vine
Derris scandens
Tao Wan Prieng

Action: Analgesic, Antispasmodic, Diuretic, Purgative

Part Used: Stem

Internal Application: The stem of the jewel vine is a diuretic and a detoxifying purgative with no laxative action. It is best used for mucous congestion, internal infections, severe colds, and dysentery, where antimicrobial action is desired without agitation of the gastrointestinal tract.

Preparation: Decoction from roasted stem.

Topical Application: A poultice from the jewel vine is applied topically to soothe muscular pain or spasms, pulled ligaments, and tendinitis.

Preparation: Mash with mortar and pestle. Apply topically to affected areas.

Caution: Jewel vine contains estrogen-like substances, and long-term use should be avoided. Those with hormone imbalances should not use this herb.

Kaffir Lime
Citrus hystix
Ma Krut

Action: Antioxidant, Antitussive, Astringent, Blood Tonic, Carminative, Emmenagogue, Expectorant, Stomachic

Taste: Sour (fruit, leaf), bitter (rind)   **Part Used:** Juice of Fruit, Rind, Leaf

Internal Application: Kaffir lime leaves are frequently used in Thai cuisine to add a tangy flavor to soups and curries. The leaf is considered to be more medicinal than the fruit, although the juice and rind can also be used. Kaffir lime leaves and fruits are one of the main ingredients used in the traditional Thai herbal compresses, as well as in the sauna. Inhaled or ingested, kaffir lime is useful for treatment of colds, congestion, and cough. Taken internally, it is a digestion stimulant which alleviates flatulence and indigestion, and is used to promote regularity in the case of blocked or infrequent menstruation. It is well known as a blood purifier, as an antioxidant with cancer-preventing properties, and is used to treat high blood pressure.

Preparation: Make decoction from rind and/or leaves. Or add juice of the fruit to hot herbal tea. See *Special Medicinal Recipes, Chapter V* for herbal tea ideas and *Chapter IV* for more information on herbal compresses.

Note: Kaffir lime is a fruit local to Thailand. Where it is not available, the common lime may be substituted. (See *Lime.*)

Lacquer Tree
Rhus verniciflua
Rac

Action: Analgesic, Antirheumatic, Astringent

Taste: Astringent   **Part Used:** Leaf

Internal Application: The lacquer tree is the source of a dark dye used traditionally for dying robes and for ink. Tea from the leaves of the lacquer tree is used traditionally to treat diarrhea and intestinal parasites such as dysentery.

Preparation: Make tea.

Topical Application: A poultice can be made to apply topically to joint pains and arthritis.

Preparation: Mash leaves with mortar and pestle. Mix with water to make paste; apply to affected area.

Lemon
Citrus limonum (synonym: Citrus limon)
Manow

Action: Adjuvant, Antiseptic, Antitussive, Astringent, Carminative, Expectorant, Refrigerant

Taste: Sour (fruit), Bitter (rind)   **Part Used:** Juice of Fruit, Rind

Internal Application: Lemon juice is a common ingredient in cold-care treatments and is frequently added to teas to complement other herbs. Lemon juice is used to treat colds, cough, headaches, fever, arthritis, and jaundice.

Preparation: Drink a half cup (125 ml) juice diluted in water, or add to hot herbal tea. Decoction may also be made by steeping rind in boiling water.

Topical Application: Lemon is also used topically and orally as an astringent and antibacterial wash for treatment of sores. It may also be used immediately on burns as a refrigerant.

Preparation: For topical use, apply juice directly to the skin. See *Herbs in Cosmetics, Chapter III*, for more information on lemon juice as an astringent.

Note: It is said that lemon is also useful in repelling snakes. Some rural Thais keep lemon wedges by the door at night to ward off these intruders.

Lemongrass
Cymbopogon citratus
Ta khrai

Action: Antiemetic, Anti-inflammatory, Antitussive, Carminative, Diaphoretic, Digestive, Diuretic, Expectorant, Refrigerant, Stomachic, Tonic

Taste: Hot and Aromatic   **Part Used:** Stem

Internal Application: The lower part of the lemongrass stalk (technically the rhizome) is white in color and possesses the strongest flavor. This part of the lemongrass is a common ingredient in Thai soups and curries. (See *Chapter III* for recipe ideas.) Lemongrass tea is used as a therapy for colds, congestion, fever, cough, sore throat and laryngitis. As a hot herb, lemongrass is also useful as a digestion stimulant in cases of flatulence, indigestion, and constipation. Lemongrass is also used to counter stomach pains, nausea, vomiting, and back pain. Lemongrass is used by Hill-Tribes as a general tonic, for bone and joint pain, and topically for sprains, bruises, and sore muscles.

Preparation: Finely chop or pound with mortar and pestle 3–4 fresh stalks; make tea. Take 3 times daily before meals.

Licorice
Glycyrrhiza glabra
Cha Aim Tead

Action:　Antitussive, Demulcent, Diuretic, Expectorant, Laxative, Pectoral, Stimulant

Taste:　Sweet　　　　　　**Part Used:**　Root

Internal Application: Licorice root is most commonly used in the Thai tradition in cold remedies, as well as for flu, cough, congestion, and fever. It is useful for soothing mucous membranes and may be used in cases of stomach pain, peptic ulcers, sore throat, laryngitis, lung disease, and bronchial infections. As a diuretic, it is also useful against infections and disorders of the bladder and kidneys, kidney stones, diabetes, and hypoglycemia. Licorice is a general stimulant, with a particular effect on the circulatory system and the heart. It increases blood pressure and stimulates the heart muscle. In the Western traditions, licorice is used as a laxative to counter flatulence and constipation and is gentle enough in small doses to be safe for children and infants.

Preparation: Tea from 1 tsp dried powdered root in 1 cup (250 ml) water.

Caution: Licorice is a hypertensive and may not be appropriate for people with high blood pressure.

Lime
Citrus aurantifolia, Citrus acida
Ma Nao

Action:　Antitussive, Appetizer, Astringent, Blood Tonic, Carminative, Digestive, Emmenagogue, Expectorant, Refrigerant, Stomachic

Taste:　Sour (fruit), Bitter (rind), Bland (root)　**Part Used:**　Juice of fruit, Rind

Internal Application: In traditional Thai herbalism, the kaffir lime is almost always preferred because of its stronger medicinal effects. However, when it is unavailable, the common lime may be used. Like the kaffir, the common lime is useful for treatment of colds, congestion, and cough. It is a digestion stimulant which alleviates flatulence and indigestion. Lime juice is considered to be a blood tonic and is used to promote regularity in the case of blocked or infrequent menstruation. The Wat Po texts mention lime leaf as a remedy for asthma, epilepsy, parasites, blood diseases, fevers, poisoning, headache, cough, mucous congestion, sore throat, and mouth sores. The juice is mentioned as a cure for cough and cold, and as an appetizer. The root is mentioned as a cure for dysentery, gonorrhea, and fever.

Preparation: For stomach discomfort and indigestion, take decoction from rind 3 times daily. See *Special Medicinal Recipes, Chapter V,* for specific remedies, and *Chapter IV* for more information on herbal compresses. For cough and cold, use juice of 1 fruit diluted in herbal tea or warm water, with honey and a pinch of salt. Sip throughout the day. Dried fruit may be sucked as a lozenge.

Long Pepper
Piper retrofractum, Piper longum, Piper chaba
Dee Plee

Action: Antitussive, Carminative, Demulcent, Digestive, Expectorant, Female Tonic, Stomachic, Tonic

Taste: Hot **Part Used:** Fruit

Internal Application: The dried unripe fruit of the long pepper (a locally occurring relative of the black pepper) is commonly used as a spice in pickling and is a popular remedy used to treat colds, cough, and congestion, as well as for stimulating digestion in the case of indigestion or flatulence. It is used to treat any type of stomachache or cramps, and is also effective against diarrhea. The fruit is a tonic for the four elements, and is used to tonify the uterus after childbirth by encouraging uterine contraction.

Preparation: Soak 1 fresh fruit in water with lemon juice and salt. For stomach discomfort or indigestion, boil 10–12 dried fruits 10–15 minutes in 1 pint (500 ml) water. Drink $1/3$ glass 3 times daily after meals.

Caution: Long pepper may be an abortifacient and should be strictly avoided by pregnant women.

Longan
Euphoria longana
Lamyai

Action: Blood Tonic, Female Tonic, Nervine, Nutritive Tonic, Sedative

Taste: Sweet **Part Used:** Fruit

Internal Application: Related to the lychee, the longan berry is one of the most celebrated fruits of Northern Thailand, and a yearly festival is held in its honor every August in the town of Lumphun. The longan is a refreshing summer fruit, and iced longan juice helps to take the edge off an over-heated day. The longan is a nutritive tonic familiar to Chinese herbalism, and a powerful tonic for the brain, senses, memory, and blood. It is especially beneficial for women post-partum, as it is beneficial for the female reproductive system. In both sexes, it is a calmative recommended for insomnia, heart palpitations, stress, anxiety, and vertigo.

Preparation: Eat fruit raw or dried, or make juice with fresh fruits.

Phyllanthus amarus, Phyllanthus niruri
Loog Thai Bai, Bahupatra

Action: Antipyretic, Antiseptic, Appetizer, Bitter Tonic, Blood Tonic, Diuretic, Hepatic, Sedative, Stomachic, Vulnerary

Taste: Bitter   **Part Used:** Whole plant

Internal Application: Loog thai bai (pronounced "lewk tye bye") is one of the most useful bitter plants in the Thai pharmacopoeia. It is very beneficial for the kidneys and liver, and is held to be an excellent daily tonic for diabetes and hypoglycemia. It has a calming effect on the circulatory system, lowering blood pressure in the case of hypertension, and relieves stress, nervousness, insomnia, and anxiety. As a bitter tonic, loog thai bai is prescribed for any type of liver disease such as hepatitis and cirrhosis, and for cases of jaundice. As an effective diuretic, it is used to treat inflamed kidneys, gall stones, prostate disease, gout, diseases of the pancreas, gonorrhea, venereal disease, excessive or frequent menstruation, as well as cases of infrequent or painful urination. Loog thai bai is also a tonic for the stomach, easing stomach pains and increasing the appetite. It is frequently prescribed in cases of fever and back pain, and has been shown to be of use as a daily tonic for blood detoxification in cases of AIDS and other blood diseases. The Wat Po texts also mention loog thai bai as a remedy for vomiting in infants, and for malaria and flatulence.

Preparation: Powder made from dried plant, taken dry or in hot water. Dosage: 1 gram. For daily consumption as a bitter tonic, make tea from roots, stalks, and leaves. Drink 3 times daily.

Topical Application: Loog thai bai may also be used topically to as an antibacterial and vulnerary for wounds, sores, inflammations, or skin infections.

Preparation: Mix powder with a small amount of water to make a paste. Apply directly to affected area.

Lotus
Nelumbo nucifera
Dok Bua

Action: Aphrodisiac, Astringent, Cardiac, Female Tonic, Nervine, Nutritive Tonic, Sedative

Taste: Aromatic (flower), oily (seed)   **Part Used:** Flower, Seed

Internal Application: The lotus is revered across Asia wherever Hinduism and Buddhism predominate, and it is the most sacred plant in Thailand. Lotus flowers can be found growing on the grounds of most temples, universities, and government buildings. They are commonly given to monks by the devout as symbols of reverence and are positioned prominently upon Buddhist altars across Thailand. The lotus is symbolic of the human soul's transmigration through life. Growing in swamps, the plant begins its life-cycle under muddy water, slowly breaking through to the surface, where it blooms. Similarly, in the Buddhist and Hindu belief system, the soul is reincarnated again and again in the "mud" of the world, until it breaks through to the surface and blooms in Enlightenment.

Lotus may be eaten in a variety of ways. Seeds are used in many traditional Thai desserts. The bulbs are sliced and added to soups and curries, or are candied and eaten with crushed ice and lotus syrup. The seed of the lotus is used in Thai medicine as a general nutritive tonic, especially during pregnancy. As part of the daily diet, the seeds are beneficial for skin, bones, muscles, and joints. Lotus seed is a cardiac tonic recommended in cases of heart disease to strengthen the heart muscle. Inhaled, the vapor of the flower calms the nervous system, promoting a clear and peaceful mind. Lotus stamen may also be taken internally as a remedy for dizziness and nervousness.

Preparation: For medicinal use, make powder by grinding dried seeds. Fresh stamens may be taken by the teaspoon, dry or in hot tea, or may be added to steam bath for inhalation. (See *Chapter IV.*)

Bridelia burmanica, Bridelia siamensis, Bridelia ovata
Makaa

Action: Anthelmintic, Cholagogue, Digestive, Laxative, Purgative

Taste: Bitter   **Part Used:** Leaf

Internal Application: Decoction of roasted Makaa leaves is taken to treat constipation. It increases production of bile, and therefore is a digestive aid. The Wat Po texts mention makaa as a detoxifying purgative for intestinal problems and parasites and as a remedy for wasting diseases, and chronic illness. It is also considered to ease difficult childbirth.

Preparation: Roast 15 fresh or dried leaves, then boil with salt. Drink in the morning or before bed.

Caution: Unroasted leaves may cause stomach pain and nausea.

Mandarin Orange
Citrus reticulata
Som Khiew Wahn

Action: Adjuvant, Antiemetic, Antioxidant, Carminative, Digestive, Expectorant, Nutritive Tonic, Stimulant, Stomachic

Taste: Bitter   **Part Used:** Rind

Internal Application: Mandarin orange is an Asian variety, similar to a tangerine, which remains green when ripe. Orange rind is a rich source of the antioxidant vitamin C. It is a tonic for energy and immunity, stimulates the senses, and is useful as an adjuvant herb in treatments for colds, nausea, flu, and digestive problems. Due to its vitamin content, mandarin rind is also a powerful antioxidant beneficial for the eyes, brain, and immune system.

Preparation: Decoction.

Mango
Mangifera indica
Mamuang

Action: Antioxidant, Blood Tonic

Taste: Sour   **Part Used:** Fruit

Internal Application: There are many varieties of mango in Thailand, some of which are eaten ripe, and others of which are considered to be best while still green. The mango fruit is high in vitamin C and is therefore an antioxidant and immunity booster. It is recommended as a blood purifier and as a part of the daily diet for the elderly, anyone with chronic disease, smokers, and those who live in polluted areas.

Preparation: Mango is eaten ripe or unripe, dipped in a mixture of salt, sugar, and cracked red chili peppers.

Mangosteen
Garcinia mangostana
Mangkhut

Action: Antirheumatic, Antiseptic, Astringent

Taste: Astringent   **Part Used:** Rind

Internal Application: One of the most popular fruits in Thailand, the mangosteen is a sweet white fleshy fruit encased in a thick purple rind. The rind is mentioned in the Wat Po texts as an astringent used to treat diarrhea, dysentery, and hemorrhoids. Powder from the rind is also traditionally used to counter food poisoning, food allergies, and arthritis.

Preparation: Decoction from dried rind of 1 fruit. Drink every 3 hours while symptoms persist. To make powder, flame-roast skin of 1 fruit; grind finely with mortar and pestle.

Topical Application: A poultice of mangosteen rind may be used topically as an astringent to cleanse cuts, wounds, and other skin infections.

Marijuana, Cannabis
Cannabis sativa, Cannabis indica

Action: Analgesic, Antiemetic, Antispasmodic, Hypnotic, Sedative, Stomachic

Taste: Toxic   **Part Used:** Leaf, Bud, Young Shoot

Internal Application: In the Thai tradition, marijuana is used mainly as an analgesic and sedative to control pain. It is well known in the Western herbal traditions as a treatment for nausea and glaucoma, and small doses are sometimes used in both systems for calming the nervous system, combating severe nausea, and stimulating the appetite.

Preparation: Eat in food, or make tea.

Caution: Marijuana has been shown to possess highly carcinogenic effects when smoked, and is therefore recommended medicinally only as a tea or powder. Marijuana also affects the balance of hormones throughout the body and should not be used on a long-term basis. Marijuana should be avoided completely by those with hormone imbalances, and by individuals attempting to conceive.

Mawaeng
Solanum trilobatum, Solanum indicum
Mawaeng Krue (*S. trilobatum*), Mawaeng Ton (*S. indicum*)

Action: Antitussive, Bitter Tonic, Diuretic, Expectorant

Taste: Bitter   **Part Used:** Fruit

Internal Application: The unripe mawaeng fruit is used as a bitter tonic and as an expectorant for treatment of cold, cough and congestion. The ripe fruit has the same properties and is additionally eaten as a treatment for diabetes and hypoglycemia. Decoction of the root is a diuretic and expectorant.

Preparation: Pound 5–10 fresh fruits with mortar and pestle. Soak in water with a pinch of salt; strain. Sip as needed throughout the day. Or chew fresh fruits slowly to extract juice. Don't swallow solid parts. The ripe or unripe fruit may also be cooked with chili or in curries.

Milk
Nom Poung

Action: Adjuvant, Demulcent, Emollient, Nutritive Tonic

Taste: Sweet   **Part Used:** Cow's milk

Internal Application: Milk is mainly used internally as an adjuvant to enhance demulcent herbal remedies. It is a nutritive tonic and may be used in preparations to counter low energy, low immunity, and emaciation, and to build strength in children, the elderly, and those convalescing from disease or injury. Milk should not be used for illnesses with excessive congestion, as it thickens mucous.

Topical Application: Powdered milk is mainly used in the Thai tradition as a topical treatment for dry or scaly skin.

Preparation: Mix with hot water to make paste; apply to skin. May also be dry-dusted on the body before sauna or steam bath (see *Chapter IV*).

Monkey Jack, Barhal
Artocarpus lakoocha
Mahaat

Action: Anthelmintic

Taste: Toxic   **Part Used:** Wood

Internal Application: Monkey jack is a potent anthelmintic used traditionally for the elimination of tapeworms and other intestinal parasites.

Preparation: Boil small pieces of wood, skimming foam that collects on top of the water. Dry foam in the sun, and crush to make a yellowish powder. Take 3 g powder before breakfast with cold water or lemon juice. Follow up 2 hours later with a laxative such as castor oil or another of the laxative herbs found in this collection.

Note: Use only cold water. If this remedy is taken with hot water, nausea or vomiting may result.

Mulberry
Morus alba, Morus nigra, Morus indica
Bai Mon

Action: Anthelmintic, Antipyretic, Antitumor, Antitussive, Aphrodisiac, Carminative, Laxative, Purgative, Sedative   **Part Used:** Bark of Root, Leaf

Internal Application: As a laxative, mulberry root bark is used to counter constipation, indigestion, and flatulence. It is prescribed for fever, cough, and in cases of anxiety, stress, or nervousness. It is also said to be an aphrodisiac. Mulberry root bark has been shown to have tumor-shrinking properties and is therefore being researched for treatment of cancer. A tea of mulberry leaves is a popular Thai tea with immune-boosting antioxidants and anticancerous alkaloids. In larger doses, it is used as a purgative to expel tapeworms and other intestinal parasites. A decoction of the leaves is diluted and used as eye drops for conjunctivitis, sties, and other eye infections.

Preparation: Tea from dried leaves, decoction of root bark, or grind dried root bark to make powder. Take 1/2 tsp dry or with hot water.

Caution: The unripe fruit of the mulberry is poisonous.

Musk
Kee Cha Mod

Action: Analgesic, Anti-inflammatory, Antitumor, Aphrodisiac, Emmenagogue, Stimulant, Tonic

Taste: Hot   **Part Used:** Musk is obtained from the glands of the male musk deer *(Moschus moschiferus).*

Internal Application: Musk is a stimulating tonic, particularly for the brain, central nervous system, and circulatory system. It is recognized as an aphrodisiac by many cultures around the world, and is therefore often used in perfumery. In the Thai tradition, musk is commonly taken medicinally as a stimulant for the nervous system and in larger doses to revive cases of fainting, unconsciousness, or coma. It is also used both internally and topically to combat tumors, to reduce swelling, and as a general analgesic.

Preparation: Musk is dried, powdered, and usually taken in pill form, ranging in dosage up to .1 gram.

Caution: Musk is an abortifacient and may cause miscarriage. It should be strictly avoided by pregnant women.

Neem
Azadirachta indica
Sadao

Action: Alterative, Anthelmintic, Antiemetic, Antihistamine, Antiparasitic, Antipyretic, Antiseptic, Astringent, Bitter Tonic, Blood Tonic, Expectorant, Stimulant, Stomachic, Vulnerary

Taste: Bitter   **Part Used:** Whole plant

Internal Application: The neem tree is a natural pharmacy in and of itself, and is prized by the Thai system, the Ayurvedic tradition of India, and indeed throughout Asia, as an essential source of herbal medicine. The bark of the stem is used as an astringent to treat dysentery and diarrhea. The bark of the root is used as an expectorant, a bitter tonic, and an antimalarial. The heartwood effectively treats nausea, vomiting, and parasites, and is used to calm chronic anxiety and stress, and delirium due to high fever. The fruit is an astringent anthelmintic which treats intestinal parasites, hemorrhoids, and malaria. The young shoots, leaves, and flowers are used as a bitter tonic for detoxification of blood, for treatment of vomiting, stomach pain, indigestion, fever, and malaria. Decoction of these parts is also a general internal antibacterial, antiviral, and diuretic used frequently treat dysentery, diarrhea, and parasites. Chewing the stems is said to stimulate the appetite, and the Wat Po texts mention the seed as a mild stimulant and as a treatment for poisoning.

Preparation: Decoction can be made from any part of the neem. Alternatively, the northern Thais make a delicious appetizer by stir-frying the flowers and leaves with chili sauce.

Topical Indication: The young stems of the neem tree are used throughout South Asia as a toothbrush. The ends of the stem are chewed until fine and stringy, and are then rubbed against the teeth and gums to cleanse and stimulate. Neem oil is used in natural toothpaste preparations and may also be used as a mouthwash or gargle on a daily basis. It is an antiseptic for mouth sores, gum disease, oral infections, and abscesses. (See mouthwash and tooth powder recipes in *Herbs in Cosmetics, Chapter III*.) Due to its antibacterial properties, the oil of the neem tree is a common additive to soap, and may also be dropped into the ear canal to treat infections. Applied to the skin, the leaf, seed, and/or oil cures fungal infections, eczema, acne and scabies, lice, ringworm, and other skin parasites, and may safely be used as a vaginal douche for infections. Hill-Tribes use neem for dermatitis, rash, and warts. Neem oil is often used in cosmetic skin preparations to enhance skin tone, elasticity, and youthfulness. It is also an effective insecticide.

Preparation: Essential neem oil may be added to fragrance-free skin lotion or to olive oil. Use 5%–10% neem oil. Neem tea for use as a mouthwash can be made with fresh stems or pure essential oil, but be sure to dilute well, as the flavor is intensely bitter. The tea may also be used as a hair rinse, vaginal douche, or skin toner. (See *Herbs in Cosmetics, Chapter III*, for additional ideas.)

Night Jasmine, Coral Jasmine
Nyctanthes arbor-tristis
Kanika

Action: Antipyretic, Appetizer, Cholagogue, Laxative, Tonic

Taste: Aromatic   **Part Used:** Whole plant

Internal Application: While not properly a species of jasmine, the night jasmine has many of the same medicinal properties as *Jasminum officinale*. The flower is used to treat fever and vertigo, and was used traditionally to make a saffron-colored dye used for monks' robes. Decoction of the stem relieves headache. The leaf is a cholagogue, stimulating appetite and enhancing digestion by increasing the production of bile. The root is a laxative and a tonic which balances the four elements.

Preparation: Mash fresh flowers, leaf, and/or root with mortar and pestle, adding a bit of water to make a paste. Strain; take liquid 1–3 times daily before meals. Flowers may also be added to sauna or steam bath (see *Chapter IV*).

Noni, Indian Mulberry
Morinda citrifolia
Yo Baan

Action: Alterative, Analgesic, Antiemetic, Anti-inflammatory, Antioxidant, Antitumor, Digestive, Emmenagogue, Nutritive Tonic, Stomachic

Part Used: Fruit

Internal Application: In Thailand, the unripe noni fruit is traditionally used as a digestive and to counter nausea and vomiting. This fruit is widely known throughout the Pacific islands, however, as a universal panacea, and its popularity is growing worldwide. Noni has been used successfully for treating colds, tuberculosis, flu, asthma, indigestion, gastritis, chronic constipation, and internal parasites, as well as for bladder, kidney, and urinary tract infections and disease. It is a rich source of vitamin C and other antioxidants, and is used as a nutritive tonic to boost the immune system. The noni fruit is also a tonic for the respiratory system, controls high blood pressure, treats diabetes and hypoglycemia, and has been shown to retard the growth of tumors and cancerous cells. In modern Thailand, it is used as a daily tonic in the treatment of cancer, HIV-AIDS, hepatitis, and other severe diseases.

Preparation: Thinly slice unripe fruit and fire roast. Decoction from 2 handfuls of roasted fruit in 1 pint (500 ml) water. Drink as necessary while symptoms persist, or take daily as a tonic. The raw fruit may also be substituted for papaya when making *Som Tam* (see recipe in *Chapter III*). The young leaves and shoots are frequently steamed and eaten with chili or added to soups and curries.

Nutgrass, Sedge Root, *Musta*
Cyperus rotundus
Ya Haew Moo

Action: Alterative, Analgesic, Anthelmintic, Antipyretic, Antispasmodic, Astringent, Carminative, Cardiac, Diaphoretic, Digestive, Diuretic, Emmenagogue, Hepatic, Stimulant, Stomachic, Tonic

Taste: Bitter   **Part Used:** Rhizome

Internal Application: Taken daily, nutgrass is a tonic for the liver and heart, a digestion stimulant, and an aid against hypertension. It is extremely useful in cases of blocked or infrequent menstruation, menstrual cramps, and PMS. In the Thai tradition, it is used to treat fevers, especially those that occur during menstruation. It is also commonly used to treat diarrhea, dysentery, stomach or intestinal cramps, irritable bowel, gastritis, indigestion, flatulence, colds, flu, and congestion.

Preparation: Pound 1 handful rhizome with mortar and pestle. Make decoction, or eat pulp with honey. Use ginger as an adjuvant.

Nutmeg
Myristica fragrans
Chan Thet

Action: Antipyretic, Antispasmodic, Aphrodisiac, Appetizer, Astringent, Blood Tonic, Carminative, Digestive, Male Tonic, Nervine, Pectoral, Sedative

Taste: Hot   **Part Used:** Wood, Seed

Internal Application: The seed kernel is properly called nutmeg, while the membrane that covers the kernel is called mace. Nutmeg is used in small quantities in Thai cuisine as an appetizer, digestive, and carminative. It is added as a spice to food to enhance assimilation of food, lessen flatulence, and correct sluggish digestion. Nutmeg is also considered to be a tonic for the blood and a sedative with muscle relaxant qualities. According to Ayurvedic tradition, nutmeg calms the mind and cures insomnia, incontinence of urine, and premature ejaculation. In larger doses, it is strongly hallucinogenic and has been used in some areas of the world as a psychoactive drug. Mace is not used medicinally by the Thais, but it is a popular condiment. Decoction of the wood is a lung and liver tonic.

Preparation: Add a pinch of nutmeg to food or tea.

Note: Use only a pinch of nutmeg at a time, and avoid overdose, as nutmeg may be fatally poisonous in large doses.

Nyang Plaamoo
Acanthus ilicifolius

Action: Antipyretic, Diuretic   **Part Used:** Root, Trunk, Leaf

Internal Application: This plant is a diuretic used to help expel kidney and bladder stones, and is also an antipyretic for fevers, especially those associated with skin symptoms such as measles, chicken-pox, and scarlet fever.

Preparation: Decoction

Topical Application: This plant is used topically for skin eruptions, boils, leprosy, and fevers.

Preparation: Poultice

Opium Poppy
Papaver somniferum (synonym: Papaveris somniferi)
Fin

Action: Analgesic, Antispasmodic, Antitussive, Astringent, Diaphoretic, Expectorant, Nervine, Sedative, Stimulant

Taste: Toxic   **Part Used:** Flower, Seed

Internal Application: While opium addiction and narcotics trafficking are two of Thailand's most pressing social problems, the opium poppy has long been held in esteem by traditional herbalists for its potent medicinal effects. Taken internally, opium is one of the most effective natural anesthetics, and it is traditionally employed to these purposes in rural Thailand where modern anesthetics are unavailable. In small doses, opium is a mild stimulant. In larger doses, it is used as a temporary calmative in severe cases of anxiety or panic attacks. Opium is also mentioned in the Wat Po texts as a very effective remedy for cough, diarrhea, dysentery, rectal bleeding, and hemorrhoids. The seeds of the poppy, commonly available commercially in the West, have an astringent effect and are taken to treat diarrhea and dysentery.

Preparation: The juice of the poppy flower head is extracted by incision. The juice is dried to make resin and is then smoked, eaten, or applied topically. The seeds of the poppy are dry-roasted and ground to a fine powder to be taken by the teaspoon.

Topical Application: A poultice of opium resin is used topically as a local analgesic for management of pain and soothing of muscle spasms. It may be applied to the temples to alleviate headache.

Caution: This herb is presented here in the context of traditional Thai herbalism. The dangers of overdose and addiction are such that the use of opium poppy is not recommended by the author of this collection.

Oroxylum
Oroxylum indicum
Phae Kaa

Action: Anti-inflammatory, Antipyretic, Antirheumatic, Antitussive, Astringent, Expectorant, Female Tonic, Stomachic, Vulnerary

Taste: Astringent   **Part Used:** Whole plant

Internal Application: Oroxylum bark tea is used traditionally as a uterine tonic after childbirth. It is also used in treatment of diarrhea, arthritis, and measles. Oroxylum seeds and bark are prescribed in cases of sore throat and cough, especially when accompanied by chills, fever, or other cold symptoms. The root, stem and bark is an antidiarrheal and a tonic for the four elements. This herb is extremely popular among the Hill-Tribes, who use it for treatment of indigestion, stomachache, inflammation, kidney and bladder disease, spleen disease, malaria, and cancer.

Preparation: Make decoction from 100 grams bark in 1¹/₂ pints (750 ml) water; take 1 tbs dose 2 times daily for 7–8 days. Or simmer 2–3 grams dried seeds in 1 pint (500 ml) water for 1 hour; strain; drink decoction in 1 day separated into 3 doses after meals. The young leaves may be eaten raw, and the green pods are sometimes added to curries to aid in digestion.

Topical Application: The Hill-Tribes apply a poultice of oroxylum to broken bones, burns, rashes, dermatitis, cuts, wounds, and muscle pain.

Caution: Oroxylum acts as an abortifacient and should be strictly avoided by pregnant mothers.

Otaheite Gooseberry, Star Gooseberry
Phyllanthus acidus
Ma-yom

Action: Antipyretic

Taste: Sour　　　　　　　　　　　　**Part Used:** Fruit

Internal Application: Otaheite gooseberries are traditionally eaten for cases of fever, chronic thirst, and measles.

Preparation: Eat fruit raw, dipped in a mix of salt, sugar, and chili. The raw leaves may be eaten as well.

Oyster
Huynarom

Action: Carminative, Digestive, Diuretic

Taste: Salty　　　　　　　　　　　　**Part Used:** Shell of Ostrea spp.

Internal Application: Ground oyster shells are a traditional treatment for kidney stones, flatulence, and indigestion. Due to the high calcium content of the shell, it is also recommended as a dietary supplement for those with bone disease or fractures.

Preparation: Oyster shell is readily available in capsule form in most vitamin and herbal supplement stores.

Pandanus, Screw Pine
Pandanus tectorius, Pandanus odoratissimus
Toey Hawm

Action: Antipyretic, Cardiac, Carminative, Digestive, Diuretic, Expectorant

Taste: Sweet　　　　　　　　　　　　**Part Used:** Root, Flower

Internal Application: The male pandanus flower is a tonic for the heart. The root is a diuretic used to help expel kidney or bladder stones. It also reduces fever, mucous congestion, and relieves indigestion and flatulence.

Preparation: Decoction.

Papaya
Carica papaya
Malakor

Action: Anthelmintic, Antioxidant, Antirheumatic, Antitumor, Cardiac, Digestive, Diuretic, Emmenagogue, Laxative, Nutritive Tonic, Stomachic, Vulnerary

Taste: Hot (seed), Sweet (fruit)   **Part Used:** Seed, Fruit, Leaf, Root

Internal Application: Papaya is a digestion stimulant which aids in assimilating food due to the large amount of the enzyme papain present in the fruit. The enzyme is so effective that, in many parts of the tropics, tough meat is soaked overnight in a marinade that contains papaya pulp or juice as a tenderizer. Papaya also contains large quantities of vitamins A and C, well known antioxidants. The fruit of the papaya is eaten both ripe and unripe (see *Som Tam* recipe in *Chapter III* for a recipe based on unripe papaya). While the unripe fruit is a digestive, the ripe fruit and the seeds are mild laxatives taken medicinally to treat constipation, indigestion, flatulence, and cramping of the intestines. Papaya seed, with a powerful spicy flavor, is also used to purge dysentery and other parasites of the gastrointestinal tract. The root is a diuretic used to treat venereal diseases such as gonorrhea. Papaya is recommended as part of the daily diet for cases of arthritis, allergies, asthma, hypertension, chronic anxiety, influenza, toothaches, and cancerous tumors. Either the seeds or the fruit may be taken as a general tonic for low immunity, low energy, chronic fatigue, and wasting diseases.

Preparation: Eat papaya fruit in the morning on an empty stomach, or take 1 tsp seeds after meals.

Topical Application: The leaf of the papaya is used topically on wounds, skin ulcers, and other sores, as it cleanses and speeds healing. Papaya rind is also used in preparations for skin and hair (see *Chapter III* for recipes).

Preparation: Bruise leaves with mortar and pestle; apply topically to affected areas.

Paracress, Spilanthes
Spilanthes acmella
Phak Khraat Hua Wan

Action: Analgesic, Antiemetic, Antipyretic, Antirheumatic, Antiseptic, Appetizer, Carminative, Digestive, Stomachic

Part Used: Whole plant

Internal Application: Paracress tea is a digestion stimulant. It is useful in cases of flatulence, nausea, and vomiting, and is also prescribed for fever, arthritis, and gout. Mixed with vinegar, it makes a mild antiseptic for mouth sores and sore throat. The stems are also chewed for toothache and are sometimes given to children with speech disorders such as stuttering. Paracress is said to cure these problems, as well as paralysis of the tongue and general weakness of the mouth.

Preparation: Tea. For toothache, stems and flowers may be pounded with a mortar and pestle, mixed with a pinch of salt, and chewed.

Peppermint
Mentha piperita, Mentha cordifolia, Mentha arvensis
Saranae

Action: Analgesic, Antiemetic, Antispasmodic, Antitussive, Aphrodisiac, Appetizer, Carminative, Cholagogue, Diaphoretic, Digestive, Expectorant, Nervine, Refrigerant, Sedative, Stomachic, Tonic

Taste: Hot and Aromatic   **Part Used:** Leaf

Internal Application: Peppermint tea is a general digestion stimulant and is the preferred treatment for stomach spasms or pains, nausea, abdominal cramps, indigestion, irritable bowel syndrome, and gastritis. Tea or inhalation is prescribed to treat cough. Peppermint has a calming effect on the nervous system, and the vapor is used with success in the treatment of nervousness, insomnia, and stress-related or migraine headaches.

Preparation: Tea or inhalation 2–3 times daily. Drink tea after meals. (For more information on inhalation, see *Chapter IV.*)

Note: *M. piperita* is preferred over the other two varieties, as its effects are stronger.

Oenanthe stolonifera
Phak Chee Lom

Action: Antiemetic, Antipruritic, Antitussive, Carminative, Diaphoretic, Purgative

Part Used: Whole plant

Internal Application: Phak chee lom is used in decoction as a carminative to treat asthma, cough, and bronchitis. It is a diaphoretic which detoxifies the skin through inducement of sweating. It is considered to be a purgative with no laxative action and is also used to counter nausea and vomiting.

Preparation: Decoction

Topical Application: This plant is used in the traditional sauna or steam bath for treatment of skin infections, allergies, and hives.

Preparation: See *Chapter IV* for more information.

Pineapple
Ananas cososus
Sapparot

Action: Anti-inflammatory, Antitussive, Blood Tonic, Diuretic, Expectorant, Female Tonic, Hepatic, Nervine, Nutritive Tonic, Stomachic

Taste: Sour   **Part Used:**   Fruit, Rhizome

Internal Application: The rhizome of the pineapple plant is a diuretic recommended for those suffering from kidney diseases, kidney stones, bladder infections, and urinary tract infections. Pineapple fruit juice is recommended for inflammatory internal diseases, diseases of the liver, and cough or cold with congestion. It is a nutritive tonic for convalescence and is said to detoxify the entire system. It is also recommended for diseases of the uterus and for post-partum tonification and strengthening of the female reproductive organs. The fruit juice is used in treatment of depression, and due to the vitamin content, has an especially beneficial effect on the brain and nervous system. The Hill-Tribes take pineapple juice to treat stomachache and use it topically on warts, rashes, and dermatitis.

Preparation: Eat fruit raw, or drink juice. Pineapple shoots and fruit are used in curries, soups, and stir-fries.

Plantain
Plantago major
Phak Kaat Nam

Action: Alterative, Antitussive, Astringent, Demulcent, Digestive, Diuretic, Expectorant, Hemostatic, Stomachic, Vulnerary

Taste: Astringent **Part Used:** Whole plant

Internal Application: The fresh juice from the whole plant is drunk as a diuretic to treat bladder or urinary tract infections and kidney stones. It is an expectorant to help clear up cough, laryngitis, sore throat, and any other respiratory problems. It soothes digestive problems, peptic ulcers, and gastritis. As an astringent, it is used to counter mucous or blood in the stool, sputum, or vaginal discharge.

Preparation: Drink 1–2 cups of fresh plantain juice daily.

Topical Application: Apply fresh juice to dermatitis, sores, wounds, insect bites, and allergic skin eruptions. Hill-Tribes use a poultice of plantain over broken bones, and chew the plant for toothache.

Plumbago, Leadwort
Plumbago zelyanica (White Leadwort), Plumbago rosea (Rose Leadwort), Plumbago indica (Indian Leadwort)
Chettamuun Phloeng Khaao (White Leadwort), Chettamuun Phloeng Daenng (Rose Leadwort, Indian Leadwort)

Action: Blood Tonic, Diaphoretic, Diuretic, Emmenagogue, Female Tonic, Stomachic

Taste: Hot **Part Used:** Root, Bark

Internal Application: As it stimulates the Fire element and warms the body, the root of either type of plumbago is used as a carminative to stimulate digestion and as a diaphoretic. The root and/or bark of the plumbago may be used to treat cases of blocked or infrequent menstruation and to increase female fertility, although it is also an abortifacient, and should never be taken during pregnancy. Plumbago is also used to detoxify the blood and is prized by some Hill-Tribes as a general longevity tonic. The root of the rose leadwort is also used to treat hemorrhoids. The aerial parts of either plant are used in treatment of kidney disease, kidney cramps, and accompanying back pain.

Preparation: Decoction.

Caution: Plumbago may cause miscarriage and should be strictly avoided by pregnant women.

Pomegranate
Punica granatum
Tubtim

Action: Alterative, Anthelmintic, Antipyretic, Astringent, Galactogogue, Refrigerant, Stomachic, Tonic

Taste: Astringent (fruit), Toxic (root bark) **Part Used:** Fruit, Root

Internal Application: Fresh pomegranate juice is an astringent and a refrigerant, and is used to lower the body's temperature in cases of fever. The rind of the pomegranate is a strong astringent used to treat diarrhea, dysentery, blood or mucous in the stool, and food poisoning. The bark of the root is effective in purging tapeworm and other intestinal parasites. The Wat Po texts mention pomegranate flowers as a tonic to improve the quality of breast milk.

Preparation: For diarrhea, prepare decoction by boiling dried rind of ¼ fruit in 1 cup (250 ml) boiling water with a pinch of quicklime. Take once or twice daily. For purgative, decoction of root bark may be taken in the morning for up to 10 days. For dysentery and chronic diarrhea, use the famous "Five Parts" recipe: young leaves, fruit, flowers, stem and root. Always use cloves with pomegranate as an adjuvant to lessen the unpleasant side effects such as headache and/or nausea that occur at proper dosage.

Topical Application: Fresh pomegranate juice may be used topically as an astringent and antifungal, or as a gargle for sore throat or mouth sores.

Preparation: The entire fruit (without the peel) may be liquefied in a blender and strained. Apply juice directly to affected areas.

Caution: Large doses of root bark may be toxic.

Pomelo
Citrus maximus
Som Oh

Action: Antipruritic

Taste: Sour   **Part Used:** Leaf

Topical Application: Pomelo fruit looks like a huge green grapefruit. The rind is thicker, and the pulp is much larger, but the flavor is similar to the pink grapefruits we know in the West. Pomelo fruit is eaten by itself or mixed with roasted garlic, onions, chili, and peanuts to make a tangy and delectable salad. Decoction of the leaf of the pomelo is used for dandruff and dry, brittle hair. It may also be added to the sauna for the same purposes.

Preparation: Decoction, steam bath, or sauna.

Pumpkin
Cucurbita moschata
Fak Thong

Action: Anthelmintic, Aphrodisiac, Diuretic, Tonic

Taste: Bland   **Part Used:** Seed, Root

Internal Application: Stewed with coconut milk and palm sugar, sautéed with red curry paste, or stir-fried with Chinese vegetables, pumpkin is a common ingredient in Thai entrees and sweets (see *Chapter III* for some recipes). The seeds are used traditionally in Eastern and Western herbalism to purge tapeworm and other intestinal parasites from the gastrointestinal tract. The Thai system holds pumpkin root to be an aphrodisiac and tonic.

Preparation: Fire roast 60 grams of seeds. Mash with mortar and pestle. Mix seeds with 500 ml water or milk. Drink 1/3 of this mixture 3 times at intervals of 2 hours. After final dose, follow up with a laxative such as castor oil or other laxative herbs found in this collection.

Note: This pumpkin is closely related to the jack-o-lantern pumpkin, *C. pepo,* which may be substituted where necessary.

Purple Allamanda, Laurel-Leaved Thunbergia
Thunbergia laurifolia
Rang Juad

Action: Antiallergic, Antipyretic, Blood Tonic, Carminative, Digestive, Diuretic

Taste: Bland   **Part Used:** Leaf

Internal Application: Purple allamanda is most commonly used in the Thai tradition as a detoxifying agent. It purifies the blood and is therefore used as an antidote to all kinds of poisonous food or chemicals. Some Hill-Tribes prescribe it for poisonous snake or insect bites. Its detoxifying properties make it the preferred treatment of hangovers, and it is prescribed daily for countering the cirrhosis associated with alcoholism. Purple allamanda is also useful in treating indigestion, flatulence, diarrhea, mucous or blood in the stool, and intestinal parasites. It is also prescribed as a remedy for fever, allergies, and asthma, and is recommended for diabetes and hypoglycemia, as it reputedly lowers blood sugar. This plant is mentioned in the Wat Po texts as a remedy for vomiting in infants, for blocked or irregular menstruation, gonorrhea, sores on the tongue and mouth, as a diuretic, and as a poultice for burns.

Preparation: Decoction.

Queen's Flower, Pride of India
Lagerstroemia speciosa
Inthanin Nam

Action: Diuretic   **Part Used:** Leaf

Internal Application: Queen's flower tea reduces blood sugar levels and is therefore good for diabetics. As a diuretic, it is also useful for irregular or painful urination, kidney and bladder stones, and venereal diseases.

Preparation: Tea

Railroad Vine, Goat's Foot Creeper
Ipomoea pes-carprae
Phakbung Talae

Action: Antipruritic   **Part Used:** Leaf

Topical Application: Railroad vine is applied topically to soothe insect bites, inflammation, allergic reactions, hives, and rashes. It also relieves the painful sting of jellyfish.

Preparation: Pound leaves with mortar and pestle. Mix with a bit of water or alcohol to make paste. (If for jellyfish stings, use distilled vinegar.) Strain, and apply liquid topically to affected areas.

Rangoon Creeper
Quisqualis indica, Quisqualis densiflora
Lep Mue Naang

Action: Anthelmintic

Taste: Toxic   **Part Used:** Seed

Internal Application: Rangoon creeper is a purgative traditionally used to expel tapeworms and other intestinal parasites. It is recommended for children, as it is not too strong for their digestive tracts.

Preparation: The kernels must be extracted from dried ripe seeds. Boil kernels in water (adult dosage 5–7 seeds, children 2–3). Strain; drink water before breakfast. Or grind dried kernels; mix with fried eggs.

Caution: Take only with cold water. Warm water may cause nausea.

Reishi Mushroom, Lingzhi Mushroom
Ganodarma lucidum
Hed Lhin-Jeu

Action: Hepatic, Tonic   **Part Used:** Mushroom caps

Internal Application: Reishi mushroom can be found in any herb market in Thailand. It has long been prized in Thai medicine, and is one of the most revered herbs in China. Reishi is traditionally used to tonify *chi* (energy), and to enhance the immune system. It is commonly used in rebuilding therapies, to strengthen and revitalize after illness, and during changes in the seasons. It has been shown to possess antiviral and antibacterial action, and to support cardiovascular and liver function. In China, it is also used to combat altitude sickness and to enhance athletic performance. This herb is also used to treat cancer, diabetes, hypoglycemia, hypertension, and chronic heart disease.

Preparation: Decoction

Safflower
Carthamus tinctorius
Dawg Kum Foy

Action: Alterative, Antirheumatic, Cardiac, Carminative, Diaphoretic, Diuretic, Emmenagogue, Laxative, Male Tonic, Tonic, Stimulant

Taste: Hot   **Part Used:**   Flower, Seed

Internal Application: Dried safflower is a tonic, especially for the heart and the circulatory and nervous systems. Because of its beneficial effect on the circulation, it is used to treat cases of male sexual dysfunction and to encourage regularity in cases of blocked, irregular, or painful menstruation. The flower is used as a calmative in cases of stress, anxiety, and panic attacks. It is also an effective therapy for colds, arthritis, and constipation. The seed is a purgative and expectorant, and may also be used to encourage menstruation and to lower cholesterol.

Preparation: Tea from 1 tsp dried flowers. Drink twice daily.

Topical Application: Safflower is used topically as an antibacterial, as well as to ease inflammation, arthritis, pinched nerves, and sciatica.

Preparation: Oil from the seeds is mixed with equal parts vegetable oil and alcohol. Massage affected parts with oil, or add to compress (see *Chapter IV*).

Salet Phangphon
Clinacanthus nutans

Action: Antipruritic   **Part Used:**   Leaf

Topical Application: A tincture of salet phangphon (pronounced "sah-let pang-pon") is used topically to soothe skin ulcers, herpes, allergic rash, hives, shingles, burns, insect and snake bites.

Preparation: Mash 10–20 fresh leaves with mortar and pestle. Soak in alcohol for 1 week, stirring daily. Strain; apply tincture as needed to affected areas. For snake or poisonous insect bite, use 20–30 leaves, pounded with alcohol. Apply paste immediately to bite for 30 minutes.

Sandalwood Tree
Adenanthera pavonina
Maklam Tah Chang

Action: Alterative, Anti-inflammatory, Antipruritic, Antipyretic, Antiseptic, Bitter Tonic, Blood Tonic, Hemostatic, Refrigerant, Sedative

Taste: Bitter   **Part Used:**   Wood, Essential oil

Internal Application: Sandalwood is taken internally to treat fever and to detoxify the blood. It is used by Hill-Tribes to revive unconscious patients and as a tonic.

Preparation: Decoction of wood.

Topical Application: Sandalwood paste is used by many in South Asia as a topical refrigerant. In many places, a small smudge is applied over the third eye or on the forehead to cool the entire body and to lessen sweating. These smudges have taken on religious symbolism in India and are used to differentiate different Hindu sects. Sandalwood paste is not used in this way in Thailand, although sandalwood oil is a frequent ingredient in soaps, shampoos, and fragrances, all of which have the same cooling effect on the body. Sandalwood may also be applied to dermatitis, herpes and infection, and inflammation of the skin.

Preparation: The Ayurvedic recipe for sandalwood paste calls for 4 oz (120 grams) sandalwood powder in 1 pint (500 ml) water. Let sit overnight. Combine with 1 pint (500 ml) coconut oil and cook without boiling over a low flame until water has evaporated.

Sarapee
Ochrocarpus siamensis (synonym *Mammea siamensis*)

Action: Blood Tonic, Cardiac, Tonic

Taste: Aromatic **Part Used:** Flower

Internal Application: The sarapee flower is used as a tonic for the heart, blood, and circulatory system. It is especially recommended as a longevity tonic for older adults.

Preparation: Drink tea, or add to sauna or steam bath.

Satinwood, Orange Jasmine, China Box Tree
Murraya paniculata
Kaew

Action: Anti-inflammatory **Part Used:** Leaf

Topical Application: A tincture of satinwood is used topically as an anti-inflammatory. It soothes sprains, joint pain, bone pain, contusions, toothaches, and swollen, painful insect and snake bites.

Preparation: Mash 15 leaves with mortar and pestle. Soak in alcohol 3–5 minutes; strain. Apply tincture to affected areas on skin or mouth.

Sea Holly
Acanthus ebracteatus
Ngueak plea mo

Action: Antiseptic, Diuretic, Tonic **Part Used:** Whole plant

Internal Application: The leaf of the sea holly is combined 2 parts to 1 with black pepper as a longevity tonic. The seed is anthelmintic. The juice is used as a hair tonic. The whole plant is a diuretic used to treat kidney and bladder stones.

Preparation: Decoction

Topical Application: The whole plant is used as a topical antibacterial.

Preparation: Poultice

Sea Salt
Glaur Talay

Action: Antiseptic, Laxative, Purgative

Taste: Salty

Internal Application: Sea salt is used in Thai medicine as a gargle for mouth sores and infections. A sea salt solution may be drunk twice daily as a laxative, to purge the digestive system of excessive mucous, and to encourage drainage of lymph. The same solution may be used as a disinfectant eyewash, gargle, nasal wash, or enema, and may be swallowed and vomited up to remove mucous or foreign matter from the stomach.

Preparation: Drink 3 tbs sea salt in 1 pint (500 ml) lukewarm water.

Sensitive Plant
Mimosa pudica, Mimosa hispida
Naiyaraap *(M. pudlica),* Rangap *(M. hispida)*

Action: Analgesic, Diuretic   **Part Used:** Whole plant

Internal Application: The whole plant is decocted and taken internally by many Hill-Tribes as a diuretic for kidney dysfunction and/or stones. Sensitive plant also is used in the Thai tradition to treat anemia, jaundice, and emaciation. The root is a remedy for dysentery. A tincture in alcohol is used to lower high blood sugar levels.

Preparation: Decoction

Topical Application: Sensitive plant is used topically for aching muscles.

Preparation: Poultice or hot compress.

Sesame Seeds
Sesamum indicum
Nga

Action: Antirheumatic, Demulcent, Emmenagogue, Emollient, Laxative, Nutritive Tonic

Taste: Oily   **Part Used:** Seed, Oil

Internal Application: In Thai medicine, sesame seeds are recommended dietary supplements for sufferers of joint problems, tooth decay, and bone weakness. Sesame promotes strength and increases body warmth and is therefore a nutritive tonic as part of the daily diet. As a demulcent, sesame seed is also taken in cases of cough, constipation, hemorrhoids, and painful or blocked menstruation.

Preparation: Eat seeds raw or dry-roasted, or use sesame oil. Seeds or oil may be added to salads, vegetables, and other dishes as an alternative to less-beneficial oils such as peanut or vegetable-based oils frequently used in Asian cuisine. (See also *Sesame Leaf Snack* recipe in *Chapter III.*)

Shorea
Shorea roxburghii
Phayom

Action: Astringent | **Part Used:** Flower

Internal Application: Shorea flowers are used to treat diarrhea, bloody stool, or other excessive discharge.

Preparation: Flowers can be eaten raw or steamed with chili sauce. They are frequently eaten with fried eggs or in the hot and sour soup called "kaeng som." Shorea is also a typical ingredient in betel-nut preparations, which are chewed as a general stimulant in many areas of South Asia.

Soap Nut, Soap Berry
Sapindus rarak
Makham Dee Khwai

Action: Antiparasitic, Antipruritic, Antipyretic, Antiseptic, Bitter Tonic

Taste: Bitter | **Part Used:** Seed, Fruit

Internal Application: The seed of the soap nut tree is traditionally used for treatment of fever and food poisoning, and is considered to be a bitter tonic. The Wat Po texts mention the pulp of the soap nut fruit as an antibacterial used in making ear drops.

Topical Application: The soap nut fruit was at one time used in South Asia as a natural soap and still is an ingredient in natural herbal soaps and shampoos. In Thailand, the soap nut is used medicinally to counter itching of the skin such as in the case of allergic reactions, hives, rashes, and dandruff. It is also used as a skin tonic and as a remedy for ringworm.

Preparation: Make decoction from 4–5 de-pitted and crushed fruits. Apply decoction to skin or scalp twice daily.

Aganonerion polymorphum
Somlom

Action: Digestive, Laxative, Stomachic

Taste: Sour | **Part Used:** Root, Leaf

Internal Application: Decoction of the root is used to treat abdominal cramps, intestinal pain, stomachache, indigestion, irritable bowel, and gastritis. The leaf has a laxative effect as well and has a tangy lemon-like flavor that tastes great in soups or curries.

Preparation: Decoction of root. Eat leaves raw or cooked. A traditional rural recipe for a delicious laxative soup calls for somlom leaves stewed with galangal, garlic, and chili peppers.

Star Anise, *Chinese Anise*
Illicium verum
Poy kak

Action: Analgesic, Antispasmodic, Antitussive, Carminative, Digestive, Emmenagogue, Expectorant, Sedative, Stomachic

Taste: Hot and Sweet   **Part Used:** Seed, Pod

Internal Application: Anise is mainly a digestive and stomachic used to counter flatulence, indigestion, irritable bowel, gastritis, and other stomach or intestinal cramping. It is gentle enough to use safely with children and infants. Star anise is a useful cold remedy for cases of dry cough, congestion, flu, and sore throat. As an expectorant, it is especially useful in cases of bronchitis, asthma, and other respiratory infections. It is an excellent remedy for insomnia and promotes regular menstruation.

Preparation: Make tea with 3–4 star-shaped pods, or 1 tsp dried seeds. Drink after meals.

Stevia, *Sweet Leaf*
Stevia rebaudiana
Yaa Wann

Action: Adjuvant

Taste: Sweet   **Part Used:** Leaf

Internal Application: This leaf is a native of Brazil and Paraguay but is currently grown widely in South East Asia and China as a sugar substitute for diabetics, hypoglycemics, and weight-conscious individuals. By weight, it is up to 300 times sweeter than sugar but has virtually no calories. Diabetics and hypoglycemics should always use stevia as a sweetener in herbal teas rather than honey or sugar, as it does not cause spikes in blood sugar.

Preparation: Use the dried and powdered leaf as you would use sugar. Alternatively, a sweetening syrup may be made by boiling stevia in a small amount of water. Use up to 1 gram per day.

Sting-Ray
Pla Kraben

Action: Female Tonic, Nutritive Tonic

Taste: Salty   **Part Used:** Tail of *Dasyatis bleekeri*

Internal Application: The meat of the sting-ray's tail is prized for its tonic properties in a way similar to the blue crab (see *Blue Crab*). It is typically eaten by children to prevent a host of childhood illnesses and by new mothers for tonification of uterus and other female reproductive organs after pregnancy.

Preparation: Eat steamed.

Sugar Apple, *Sweet Sop, Custard Apple*
Annona squamosa
Noinae

Action: Antiparasitic

Taste: Toxic (leaf, seed), Sweet (fruit)   **Part Used:** Leaf, Seed

Internal Application: A popular fruit in northern Thailand, the sugar apple is used medicinally for treatment of lice.

Preparation: Grind 8–12 seeds or 15 g fresh leaves to a powder. Mix 1 part powder with 2 parts coconut oil. Apply to hair, and wrap with cloth. After a half hour, wash thoroughly. Repeat once a day for 2–3 days to kill lice and eggs. This preparation may also be used to kill ringworm and other skin parasites.

Caution: This preparation is toxic and is an irritant to the eyes and other mucous membranes. Use with care.

Sugar Cane
Saccharum spp.
Oi Daeng

Action: Adjuvant, Antitussive, Demulcent

Taste: Sweet   **Part Used:** Various types of sugar and their uses follow

Internal Application: Sugar cane (S. officinarum) is commonly available from vendors in the streets of South Asia. Whereas in India, traveling cane-presses allow a thirsty visitor to enjoy a fresh-squeezed glass of juice, in Thailand, iced sugar cane is sold in bite-sized chunks. The cane is chewed, and the woody pulp is spat out when the juice has been extracted. Any way it is eaten, there are few things more pleasurable on a hot sticky day than fresh sugar cane.

Traditionally, sugar is added as an adjuvant to herbal teas to soothe the throat and to make the taste more palatable. Different types of sugar will be added depending on the symptoms. Fresh sugar cane juice is added to treat fever, sore throat, cough, congestion, bladder infections, urinary tract infections, low energy, low immunity, chronic disease, chronic fatigue, and emaciation. Raw, unrefined sugar is added to herbal teas that treat fever and lymph problems. Rock sugar is added to treatments for fevers, colds, and sore throat. Juice of the black sugar cane *(S. sinense)* is a diuretic used in remedies for kidney disorders and venereal diseases.

Preparation: Sugar cane juice can be extracted with a press specifically made for that purpose or can be bought in cans or bottles at Asian groceries. If using granulated sugar, only use raw, unrefined sugar (such as Turbinado or "Sugar in the Raw"™). Never use common white or brown sugar, which have no medicinal qualities. For medicinal use of black sugar cane, take juice of 70–90 g fresh cane or 30–40 g dried, 3 times daily before meals.

Sugar Palm
Arenga spp.
Dtao

Action: Adjuvant, Demulcent

Taste: Sweet **Part Used:** Sap

Internal Application: Palm sugar, also known as jaggery, is added as an adjuvant to herbal teas that treat colds, sore throat, and congestion.

Sulfur
Gum Matun

Action: Antiparasitic

Taste: Toxic

Topical Application: Sulfur paste is applied topically to fungal infections, acne, ringworm, scabies, and other skin parasites. It is also commonly used in Thailand to treat mange on dogs.

Preparation: Apply paste topically on affected areas. Powder may be applied dry or with petroleum jelly.

Tako Naa
Diospyros rhodocalyx

Action: Antiseptic, Tonic **Part Used:** Stem

Internal Application: A relative of the ebony tree, tako naa is used to balance the four elements, as a longevity tonic, a mouthwash for toothache and gum disease, and a treatment for vaginal discharge.

Preparation: Decoction, with a pinch of salt.

Tamarind
Tamaridus indica
Ma Khaam

Action: Anthelmintic, Antipyretic, Antiseptic, Astringent, Blood Tonic, Carminative, Digestive, Expectorant, Female Tonic, Laxative, Nutritive Tonic, Purgative, Refrigerant, Stimulant, Vulnerary

Taste: Sour (fruit, leaf, bark), Oily (seed) **Part Used:** Whole plant

Internal Application: Tamarind is a common ingredient in Thai cuisine. The pulp of the fruit is cooked and added to soups and curries for flavor. The flowers, fruit, and young leaves are eaten in soups and curries. Unripe fruit is also candied and sold by street vendors coated with sugar, salt, and red chili flakes.

The fresh juice of the tamarind is the Thai equivalent of our prune juice and is a favorite remedy for constipation and fever. It is considered to be a blood purifier and is recommended for pregnancy and post-partum. Tea made from the young leaves and pods of the tamarind is a laxative and is used to treat colds and fevers. The flowers are said to lower blood pressure, and the bark is an astringent remedy for diarrhea and fever. The seeds of the tamarind are used as a purgative to expel tapeworms and other intestinal parasites, and are also recommended as a tonic for health, strength, and vigor.

Preparation: Eat 70–150 grams of fruit-pulp raw, or prepare juice by boiling pulp in water with a pinch of salt for 10–20 minutes. May be drunk hot or iced as needed. For purgative effect, dry-roast 30 seeds; soak in water until soft; eat. For colds and fevers, tea is made by steeping leaves.

Topical Application: The leaves of the tamarind are also frequently used topically to treat skin ulcers and sores. The juice and decoction of the bark are both useful astringents for general antiseptic treatment of the skin and are frequently applied directly to oily or infected skin before sauna or steam bath. (See *Chapter IV* for more information.)

Preparation: Mash leaves with mortar and pestle. Apply as poultice to affected areas.

Thai Caper
Capparis micracantha
Ching-chee

Action: Antiseptic, Antipyretic, Bronchodilator, Carminative, Stomachic

Taste: Bitter   **Part Used:** Root, Stem, Leaf

Internal Application: The root of the Thai caper is used as a carminative, a stomachic, and a bronchodilator. The root and leaf are used to treat asthma, chest pain, skin disease and chicken pox, measles, and other fevers with symptoms on the skin. The Wat Po texts mention the Thai caper as a remedy for smallpox, delirium, poisoning, and eye diseases.

Preparation: Decoction

Topical Application: Decoction of the root may be used topically as an antibacterial. The leaf relieves muscle cramps.

Preparation: Poultice

Thao Yaanaang
Tiliacora triandra

Action: Analgesic, Antipyretic   **Part Used:** Root, Leaf

Internal Application: This herb is used in the Thai tradition to treat fevers. It is used by Hill-Tribes for sprains, bruises, sore muscles, and post-delivery to lessen pain and promote healing.

Preparation: Decoction. Drink 3 times daily.

Thong Phan Chang
Rhinacanthus nasutus

Action: Anthelmintic, Antiparasitic, Antipyretic, Antiseptic, Blood Tonic, Diuretic, Laxative, Pectoral

Taste: Toxic   **Part Used:** Root, Leaf, Stem

Internal Application: Thong phan chang (pronounced "tong pan chang") is used to treat fevers, sore throat, colds, and lung diseases such as bronchitis and tuberculosis. It lowers blood pressure and is therefore effective treatment for hypertension. Tea made from this herb has a laxative effect, is held to help back pain, and is useful to encourage passing of gallstones. The Wat Po texts recommend the leaf as a diuretic, laxative, and anthelmintic, and as a detoxifying remedy for fever, blood poisoning, skin disease, and cancer. It is said that thong phan chang must be collected between sunset and sunrise because sunlight destroys the potency of the plant.

Preparation: Tea or decoction.

Topical Application: A tincture made of thong pan chang leaves is used topically as a treatment for bacterial and fungal skin infections, rashes, ringworm, and other skin parasites.

Preparation: Pound leaves with mortar and pestle. Soak in alcohol for 7 days. Apply tincture topically to affected areas 3–4 times daily. Continue application for 1 week after ringworm has disappeared.

Ti Plant, Cordyline
Cordyline fruticosa
Maak phu maak mia

Action: Antirheumatic, Astringent, Hemostatic

Taste: Bland   **Part Used:** Leaf, Bud, Young Shoot

Internal Application: The ti plant is an astringent with a wide range of applications. It is a hemostatic, used traditionally to stop bleeding in cases of bloody vomit, stool, or urine. It is also employed to stop the coughing of blood associated with tuberculosis, to halt excessive menstruation, and to curtail internal bleeding of the organs, bruises, contusions, and hematoma. The ti plant may also be used for treatment of diarrhea, dysentery, arthritis, fever, and measles. As a gargle, it is effective against tooth and gum disease, bleeding gums, and halitosis.

Preparation: Tea

Tongkat Ali
Eurycoma longifolia
Plaa Lai Phueak

Action: Antiparasitic, Antipyretic, Antitussive, Aphrodisiac, Bitter Tonic, Male Tonic, Stimulant

Taste: Bitter   **Part Used:**   Root

Internal Application: Traditionally, tongkat ali is used in Thai herbalism for treatment of colds, cough, fever, and low immunity. In other areas of Southeast Asia, it is used in a manner similar to ginseng as a male potency enhancer and aphrodisiac. The Wat Po texts mention the root as a remedy for poisoning, fever, dysentery, sunstroke, internal infections, tuberculosis, and as a topical application for skin parasites.

Preparation: Decoction. Drink morning and evening.

Toothbrush Tree, **Siamese Rough Bush**
Streblus asper
Khoi

Action: Analgesic, Antiparasitic, Antipyretic, Antiseptic, Antitumor, Appetizer, Astringent, Carminative, Digestive, Laxative, Tonic

Taste: Toxic **Part Used:** Leaf, Stem, Wood

Internal Application: The toothbrush tree seed is a longevity tonic for the four elements. It is also a carminative and appetizer, used to stimulate digestion and combat flatulence. The bark of the stem has antidiarrheal and antipyretic properties, and is often used to combat dysentery and other cases of diarrhea accompanied by fever. Infusion of the toothbrush tree leaf is a laxative and is also taken to treat all varieties of bone disease. The heartwood is traditionally dried, cut into small pieces, wrapped in dried banana leaves, and smoked for treatment of inflamed nasal passages.

Preparation: Decoction

Topical Application: The toothbrush tree, as its name would suggest, is a popular traditional remedy for tooth and gum disease. It is also applied topically to kill ringworm and other skin parasites. Another common usage is for topical treatment of hemorrhoids.

Preparation: For application to the mouth, make decoction by boiling a handful of bark with water and a pinch of salt; gargle 3–4 times daily. Or, make powder from dried bark; brush teeth and gums with powder. For application to the skin, mash fresh or dried bark with mortar and pestle. Mix with hot water to make paste; apply to affected areas. For hemorrhoids, mix paste with oil, cook. Let cool, and apply to affected area.

Note: This plant has recently been shown to have antitumor properties. Although it is not traditionally used to treat this disease, toothbrush tree is currently being studied as a treatment of cancer.

Turmeric
Curcuma longa
Khamin

Action: Alterative, Analgesic, Anthelmintic, Anti-inflammatory, Antipruritic, Antirheumatic, Antiseptic, Antitussive, Astringent, Blood Tonic, Carminative, Cholagogue, Digestive, Emmenagogue, Hepatic, Stomachic, Tonic, Vulnerary

Taste: Hot **Part Used:** Rhizome, Leaf

Internal Application: Turmeric is related to ginger and galangal, and shares some of the properties of these plants. Turmeric is used as a digestive stimulant and is often used as an adjuvant with preparations for gastrointestinal complaints, as it aids in treatment of flatulence, peptic ulcers, indigestion, irritable bowel, and gastritis. It is said to lower blood sugar and is therefore used for diabetes and hypoglycemia. Turmeric is also a remedy for cough, arthritis, chronic back pain, and painful or blocked menstruation. Turmeric leaves may be used as an antidote for food poisoning and for treatment of hepatitis, as it has a detoxifying effect on the blood, digestive tract, and liver, and regulates the body's secretion of hormones.

Preparation: Decoction from fresh rhizome or fire-roasted leaves. Drink after meals. The rhizome can also be dried and powdered. Take 500 mg powder with honey 4 times daily, with meals and before bed. Juice can also be extracted from the fresh rhizome. Young shoots and flowers are sometimes steamed and eaten with chili sauce.

Topical Application: The turmeric rhizome relives itching and swelling, and has a slight antiseptic effect. It therefore can be used topically on insect bites, rashes, allergic reactions, hives, and superficial wounds. It is also used as an anti-inflammatory for bruises and sprains.

Preparation: Mash fresh rhizome with mortar and pestle, or use powder. Mix with small amount of water to make paste; apply to affected areas.

Turkish Rhubarb, Chinese Rhubarb
Rheum palmatum

Action: Alterative, Anthelmintic, Antiemetic, Antipyretic, Antiseptic, Astringent, Cardiac, Carminative, Cholagogue, Emmenagogue, Laxative, Nervine, Purgative, Stimulant, Stomachic

Taste: Astringent   **Part Used:**   Root, Stem

Internal Application: Turkish rhubarb is well known in Eastern and Western herbalism. In large doses, it is an effective laxative, used traditionally in Thailand for treatment of constipation and flatulence and for detoxification of the colon. In lesser doses, Turkish rhubarb is used as an astringent to treat diarrhea and as a hemostatic to stop internal bleeding, bloody vomit, blood-shot eyes, and hemorrhoids. It is considered to be beneficial for the heart and brain, and is a stimulant for the production of bile. Rhubarb is also used in Western herbalism to treat nausea and blocked or irregular menstruation.

Preparation: Make powder from dried roots, stalks. Take 1 tsp dose for laxative; $1/4$ tsp dose for other complaints. Use $1/4$ tsp ginger or licorice as adjuvant to prevent stomach cramping.

Caution: While the roots and stalks of most rhubarb are edible, the leaves are poisonous.

Wan Maha Kan
Gynura pseudochina

Action: Anti-inflammatory, Antiparasitic, Antipruritic, Antipyretic

Part Used: Leaf, Root

Internal Application: The root of the wan maha kan is taken as a remedy for fever.

Preparation: Decoction

Topical Application: The fresh leaves are used topically for treatment of eczema, herpes, insect bites, scabies, lice, and skin inflammation.

Preparation: Pound leaves with mortar and pestle, adding a small amount of water to make a paste. Apply to affected areas 3–4 times daily as needed.

Water Mimosa, Neptunia
Neptunia plena, Neptunia oleracea
Pak Kachad

Action: Antipyretic

Taste: Bland   **Part Used:** Young Leaf and Stem

Internal Application: The water mimosa is a type of watercress commonly eaten in Thai salads and soups. It is used medicinally as a detoxifier to treat fever, food poisoning, and severe allergic reactions. It has also been shown to have some anti-tumor properties, and is being researched for its use as an anticarcinogen.

Preparation: The young leaves and stems are eaten raw, lightly steamed, or fried with chili sauce.

Wild Pepper Leaf
Piper sarmentosum
Chaa phluu

Action: Analgesic, Antispasmodic, Carminative, Digestive, Expectorant, Stomachic

Taste: Hot   **Part Used:** Leaf

Internal Application: The wild pepper leaf is a hot herb used traditionally to stimulate digestion, to treat flatulence, indigestion, diarrhea, and dysentery, and to ease bloated stomach, abdominal discomfort, and symptoms of irritable bowel and gastritis. It is also employed as a cold remedy, especially in the case of severe lung congestion.

Preparation: Tea

Topical Application: The wild pepper leaf is well known as a muscle relaxant and is frequently applied to aches, pains, and sore muscles.

Preparation: Apply as poultice, or use in hot compress. (See *Chapter IV* for more information.)

Woolly Grass, Imperata
Imperata cylindrica
Yaa Khaa

Action: Antipyretic, Astringent, Diuretic, Hemostatic

Taste: Sweet   **Part Used:** Root

Internal Application: Woolly grass is used primarily as a hemostatic in the treatment of blood in the vomit, urine, or phlegm. It is also used for its diuretic properties in the treatment of fevers, urinary tract infections, kidney disease and stones, cystitis, blood in the urine, and vaginal discharge. The Hill-Tribes use this grass for genital, urinary, kidney, or bladder problems, kidney and gallbladder stones, sexually transmitted diseases, and topically on acne or skin infections.

Preparation: Decoction from 40–50 grams fresh root. Take 75 ml dose 3 times daily before meals.

Ylang-Ylang, Perfume Tree
Canaga odorata
Magrut

Action: Blood Tonic, Cardiac, Diuretic

Taste: Aromatic **Part Used:** Flower, Leaf, Wood

Internal Application: Ylang-ylang flower is a tonic for the heart and is used traditionally to treat dizziness and fainting spells. It is a tonic for the blood, and it balances the four elements. The leaf and wood are diuretic.

Preparation: Make tea from fresh or dried flowers, or add flowers to sauna or steam bath. (See *Chapter IV.*)

Zedoary
Curcumin zedoaria
Khamin Oi

Action: Adjuvant, Antiemetic, Antipryretic, Antiseptic, Astringent, Stomachic

Taste: Hot **Part Used:** Rhizome

Internal Application: Related to turmeric, zedoary is used for similar purposes. It is effective against nausea, vomiting, intestinal cramps, irritable bowel, gastritis, and diarrhea, and is often added as an adjuvant to laxative herbs due to its soothing effect on the stomach. It is also effective against fever and is used by Hill-Tribes for dysentery.

Preparation: Decoction

Topical Application: Zedoary is a topical antiseptic used in the Thai tradition and by Hill-Tribes on cuts, wounds, and insect bites.

Preparation: Mash with mortar and pestle; make poultice, or add to compress. (See *Chapter IV.*)

Zerumbet Ginger
Zingiber zerumbet
Ka Thue

Action: Analgesic, Antiemetic, Antirheumatic, Stomachic

Taste: Hot **Part Used:** Rhizome

Internal Application: Zerumbet ginger has many of the same properties as common ginger, but to a lesser degree. It is used traditionally to treat stomach pain and cramping, as well as food poisoning or allergy, nausea, and vomiting. It can be used successfully to treat irritable bowel, gastritis, and indigestion.

Preparation: Decoction from fresh fire-roasted rhizome. Young shoots and flowers also may be eaten raw or steamed with chili sauce.

Topical Application: A tincture of Zerumbet ginger is applied topically to soothe arthritis pains. With massage, it is said to give especially good results.

Preparation: Soak 2 handfuls of the chopped rhizome in alcohol. Apply as needed with massage, or use hot compress (see *Chapter IV*).

Appendices

STUDYING IN THAILAND

As alternative and complementary medicine become increasingly popular at home, many Westerners are traveling to Asia to receive traditional instruction from the source. The traditional medicine institute of Bangkok's Wat Po temple remains one of the most popular schools of Thai massage among Thais, and the herbal medicine school at this temple is recognized as the most prestigious in the country. At present, however, I know of no formal English-language courses on Thai herbalism in Thailand. Many massage schools include in their curriculum an introduction to the use of herbal compress, though, and the truly dedicated can learn more through private instruction.

Chiang Mai

Chiang Mai is renowned throughout Thailand, among locals and travelers alike, as the place to go for English-language instruction in all aspects of traditional Thai medicine. Chiang Mai is the capital of Thailand's northwestern region of Lan Na and has always been a popular destination for foreign visitors. Erected on the Ping River in 1296, the city historically linked the Silk Road to Southeast Asia and long served as a cultural and commercial hub for merchant caravans from the Muslim community in southern China, the Indian-influenced kingdoms of Burma, the Khmers in Cambodia, and the Theravadin Buddhist Siam, in Central Thailand. In modern times, beautiful temples, bustling markets, and a thriving business in mountain trekking has earned Thailand's second city the reputation of a must-see among high-budget vacationers and backpackers alike. Opportunities abound for travelers interested in studying Buddhism, teaching English, or volunteering with the area's numerous Non Government Organizations (NGOs).

Perhaps the best short course on traditional massage can be found at Lek Chaiya Massage, in the main tourist section of town. As a former director of the prestigious Association of Northern Herbs, and with over 40 years of massage experience, "Mama" Lek has impeccable credentials and a well-respected style. Although she does not speak much English, Lek Chaiya has several employees who serve as both assistant teachers and translators. Instruction is both by demonstration and hands-on practice, and covers topics from acupressure points and energy meridians to herbal compresses and other therapies. Mama Lek's son, Tananan Willson, runs a medicinal tea bar below her studio, with an extensive menu of Thailand's favorite herbal remedies. For any who are interested in pursuing the study of traditional Thai massage and herbal medicine in the country of its origin, I could not recommend Lek Chaiya's school more highly.

Lek Chaiya Massage, 25 Rajadamnoen Rd., Muang Chiang Mai 50200
Web site: www.NerveTouch.com

Chiang Mai's Foundation of Shivagakomarpaj Traditional Medicine Hospital is, according to many, Thailand's premier massage school. Although the course barely touches upon herbs, it does feature a comprehensive introduction to the theory and practice of Thai medicine. The foundation's ten-day course is one of the best offered on this subject for beginners and professionals alike. Upon completion of ten days, a certification exam is given (although this certificate is not recognized in most countries). Graduates of the foundation are able to continue their education by volunteering as assistant teachers with subsequent courses, and in theory, a graduate who completes three months of volunteer work with students could apply for a position in the hospital's massage facility as a full- or part-time practitioner.

Shivagakomarpaj Traditional Medicine Hospital, 78/1 Wuolai Rd. (Across
from Old Chiang Mai Cultural Center), Chiang Mai 50100

Another massage school worth mentioning is the International Training Massage School, or ITM. Well known among backpacker circles, this school offers five-day tourist courses at a bargain price. Progressive levels of training are offered, from "Introduction" to "Teacher Training," although again, the certificates are not recognized either in Thailand or abroad. The director, Chongkol Setthakorn, has been an effective publicist and has been responsible in part for the recent rise in the popularity of Thai massage among Western practitioners of alternative medicine.

International Training Massage, 17/7 Morakot Rd, Hah Yaek Santitham,
Chiang Mai, 50300
Web site: www.InfoThai.com/ITM

Although each of these schools offers an introductory course, each teaches its own particular style of healing, and it is possible to attend all three institutions without too much repetition. There are many other schools and renowned private instructors in the Chiang Mai area, and further afield in Chiang Rai as well. English-language courses are also offered in many of the area's massage parlors, although the serious student should be aware that these schools are not always reputable. No matter which of Chiang Mai's various schools one chooses, however, the student invariably finds the educational experience to be a uniquely penetrating glimpse into Thailand's lively cultural mix. Chiang Mai's large number of massage schools offer students the chance to hone their skills and broaden their practice over a longer period of time in what still remains one of Thailand's most colorful cities.

For more information on travel to the area, refer to Chiang Mai's premiere on-line magazine at: www.chiangmai-chiangrai.com.

THAI HERBALISM COURSES AND SUPPLIERS IN THE U.S.

In the interests of promoting Thai medicine in the U.S., I offer certification courses and seminars on Thai massage, herbalism, and cuisine at various locations throughout the year. My web site includes a correspondence course based on this book, information on upcoming courses, and links to other organizations involved with Southeast Asian culture.

Tao Mountain School of Traditional Thai Massage and Herbal Medicine, 300 Rambling Rd., Ruckersville, VA 22968
Tel: (434)882-2279   Email: info@TaoMountain.org
Web Site: www.TaoMountain.org

I also maintain a website which provides a resource for procuring difficult to find Thai herbs and products discussed in this book. All of the products I distribute are grown or made in the hills of the Chiang Mai-Chiang Rai region of northern Thailand, and each purchase helps to promote the local village economies.

Visit us on-line at: *www.Thai-herbs.com*

HERBAL MEDICINE CONTACTS IN THE U.S.

The following is a list of some other herbal suppliers and organizations dedicated to quality and reliability, and I recommend the reader use these resources in procuring herbs. Although these are not specifically distributors of Thai herbs, many of the herbs in this collection can be found through the following companies. Further resources can be found through the American Herbalists Guild (see next page).

The Herb Shoppe, 4372 Chris Greene Lake Rd, Charlottesville, Virginia 22911
Tel: (434)973-1700   Email: herbshoppe@firstnetva.com
Web Site: www.HealingHerbShoppe.com

Mountain Rose Herbs, P.O. Box 2000, Redway, CA 95560
Tel: (800)879-3337   Web Site: www.MountainRoseHerbs.com

Plant-It Herbs, P.O. Box 851, Athens, OH 45701
Tel: (740)662-3413   Web Site: PlantItHerbs.com
(Specializing in live plants and Chinese herbs)

Richter's, #357 Highway 47, Goodwood, Ontario, Canada L0C 1A0
Tel: (905)640-6677   Web Site: www.Richters.com

The Herbarium, 264 Exchange St., Chicopee, MA 01013
Tel: (413) 598-8119   Web Site: www.TheHerbarium.com

The American Herbalists Guild

Although there is a long-standing tradition of officially recognized herbalism in Asia and Europe, herbal medicine is currently in a state of limbo in the U.S. While there are a few organizations attempting to regulate the market and protect patients in the process, at this point in time herbalism is a new field of knowledge, notable both for its astronomical growth and inconsistent practices. One organization that is strongly pushing for regulation of herbalism in the U.S. is the American Herbalists Guild. The only voluntary peer-review organization for American herbalists, the AHG is committed to the following missions:

1. To form a professional organization to develop, promote, and maintain levels of excellence in herbalism, including individual and planetary health.

2. To strengthen and further the network of support and communication between herbalists.

3. To foster high levels of ethics and integrity in all areas of herbalism.

4. To integrate herbalism into community health care.

5. To promote cooperation between herbalists and other health care providers, encompassing traditional wisdom and knowledge, as well as current medical models.

6. To establish and maintain standards of education for the

professional practice of herbalism.

7. To promote an ecologically healthy environment and to increase awareness concerning the interdependence of all life, especially the plant–human relationship.

8. To serve as a liaison that interfaces with other professional associations and regulatory agencies.

9. To promote further research, education, and study of herbal medicine.

Further information can be acquired by contacting the AHG directly:

American Herbalists Guild, 1931 Gaddis Rd., Canton, GA 30115
Tel: (770)751-6021   Fax: 770-751-7472
Web Site: www.AmericanHerbalistsGuild.com

HERBAL MEDICINE CONTACTS IN EUROPE

The practice of herbalism is more well established in many European countries than in the U.S., which means that there are more organizations regulating the trade. While it would be impossible to list them all, most organizations maintain web sites and can easily be found through any search engine. Here are some of the more well-known organizations.

National Institute of Medical Herbalists

Founded in 1864 by English herbalists, the NIMH is possibly the most important herbalists' organization in the U.K. The NIMH publishes the *European Journal of Herbal Medicine* and maintains a web site with up-to-date research bulletins and other resources. The members database lists practitioners across the U.K. that adhere to the NIMH's detailed code of ethics.

National Institute of Medical Herbalists, 56 Longbrook Street, Exeter EX4 6AH, U.K.
Tel: +44 (0) 1392 426022   Fax: +44 (0) 1392 498963
E-mail: nimh@ukexeter.freeserve.co.uk
Web Site: www.nimh.org.uk

The Herb Society

Another well known herbal association based in the U.K. Their mission statement states, "The Herb Society aims to increase the understanding, use, and appreciation of herbs and their benefit to health." The Herb Society publishes the journal *Herbs* and maintains a web site with useful resources for herbalists.

The Herb Society, Sulgrave Manor, Sulgrave, Banbury, OX17 2SD, U.K.
Web Site: www.herbsociety.co.uk

European Herbal Practitioners Association

A politically active group representing herbalists throughout Europe. The association's mission is to raise standards of training and promote regulation of herbalism throughout the E.U.

European Herbal Practitioners Association, 45A Corsica Street, London N5 1JT, U.K.
Web Site: www.euroherb.com

Herbal Suppliers

The following companies offer Asian herbs for sale in U.K., and shipping throughout Europe.

East-West Herbs Ltd, Langston, Priory Mews, Kingham, Oxon. OX7 6UP
Tel: 01608 658862

Herbs and Helpers, 6 Butts Fold, Cockermouth, Cumbria, CA13 9HY
Tel: 01900 826392   Web Site: www.herbalmedicineuk.com

Herbal Medicine Contacts in Australia and New Zealand

National Herbalists Association of Australia, 33 Reserve Street, Annandale, NSW 2038
Tel: (02) 9560 7077   Fax: (02) 9560 7055
Web Site: www.nhaa.org.au

New Zealand Association of Medical Herbalists, P.O. Box 15313 , Tauranga, New Zealand
Web Site: www.nzamh.org.nz

Bibliography and Further Reading

THAI MEDICINE

There are very few books that have been written on traditional Thai medicine, and those that have been published are predominantly academic works only available in Thailand. The following books, booklets, and articles, most of which can be found at the National Library in Bangkok, have been invaluable in the preparation of this present collection. Much of the material presented here first appeared in one of these works:

Anderson, Edward F. *Plants and People of the Golden Triangle: Ethnobotany of the Hill Tribes of Northern Thailand.* Portland, OR: Dioscorides Press, 1993.

Brun, Viggo and Trond Schumacher. *The Traditional Herbal Medicine of Northern Thailand.* Bangkok: White Lotus, 1994.

Jacquat, Christiane. *Plants from the Markets of Thailand.* Bangkok: Editions Duang Kamol, 1990.

McMakin, Patrick D. *Flowering Plants of Thailand: A Field Guide.* Bangkok: White Lotus, 2000

Ministry of Commerce and Communications. *Some Siamese Medicinal Plants exhibited at the Eighth Congress of Far Eastern Association of Tropical Medicine.* Bangkok: Botanical Section, Ministry of Commerce and Communications, 1930.

Mulholland, Jean. "Ayurveda, Congenital Disease and Birthdays in Thai Traditional Medicine." *Journal of the Siam Society.* 76 (1988): 174–82.

Mulholland, Jean. *Medicine, Magic, and Evil Spirits.* Canberra: The Australian National University, 1987.

National Identity Board. *Medicinal Plants of Thailand Past and Present.* Bangkok: National Identity Board, 1991.

Pecharaply, Daroon. *Indigenous Medicinal Plants of Thailand.* Bangkok: Department of Medical Sciences, Ministry of Public Health, 1994.

Ratarasarn, Somchintana. *The Principles and Concepts of Thai Classical Medicine.* Bangkok: Thai Khadi Research Institute, Thammasat University, 1986.

Saralamp, Promjit et al. *Medicinal Plants in Thailand, Vol. 1–2.* Bangkok: Department of Pharmaceutical Botany, Mahidol University, 1996, 1997.

Thai Pharmaceutical Committee. *Thai Herbal Pharmacopoeia.* Bangkok: Department of Medical Sciences, Ministry of Public Health, 1995.

Additional valuable information on traditional herbal preparation and dosage is available from the Research & Development Institute of the Government Pharmaceutical Organization, located in Bangkok, which generously shares its on-line herbal database freely in the interests of promoting traditional medicine in Thai villages. I am much indebted to this organization for allowing me to use their information in compiling this collection. The RDI can be reached at:

Research and Development Institute, Government Pharmaceutical Organization, 75/1 Rama VI Road, Rajtevi, Bangkok 10400
Web Site: www.rdi.gpo.or.th

THAI MASSAGE

The following books deal with the history, theory, and practice of Thai massage. They may be of interest to the Thai herbalist, as they deal with acupressure points, medical theory, and the history of traditional Thai healing.

Asokananda (Harald Brust). *The Art of Thai Traditional Massage.* Bangkok: Editions Duang Kamol, 1990.

Asokananda (Harald Brust). *Thai Traditional Massage for Advanced Practitioners.* Bangkok: Editions Duang Kamol, 1996.

THAI CUISINE

The culinary recipes reproduced in this book come from Chef Somphon of the Chiang Mai Cookery School, whose marvelous cookbook is available on-line at *www.thaicookeryschool.com.* I highly recommend his short courses on Thai cuisine as a wonderful introduction to Thai herbs and spices.

AYURVEDA

Since many of the roots of Thai medicine lie in the Ayurvedic traditions of India, readers of this book may find the following titles to be helpful in gaining a fuller understanding of South Asian herbalism. Most of the information on Ayurvedic traditions presented in this book comes from David Frawley's *The Yoga of Herbs,* however all of the following are helpful titles:

Balz, Rodolphe. *The Healing Power of Essential Oils.* Twin Lakes, WI: Lotus Press, 1996.

Frawley, David. *Ayurvedic Healing: A Comprehensive Guide.* Delhi: Motilal Banarisidass Publishers, 1989.

Frawley, David. *The Yoga of Herbs.* Twin Lakes, WI: Lotus Press, 1993.

Miller, Dr. Light and Dr. Bryan Miller. *Ayurveda and Aromatherapy.* Twin Lakes, WI: Lotus Press, 1995.

Ranade, Dr. Subhash. *Natural Healing Through Ayurveda.* Twin Lakes, WI: Lotus Press, 1999.

WESTERN HERBALISM

Information on the Western traditions for this collection has been obtained from the following sources:

Grieve, Maud. *A Modern Herbal.* Eugene, OR: Mountain Rose Herbs, 1981. (This book is available in on-line format at www.botanical.com)

Lust, John. *The Herb Book.* New York: Benedict Lust Publications, 2001.

Tierra, Dr. Michael. *The Way of Herbs.* Pocket Books, 1998.

CHINESE HERBALISM & TCM

Information on traditional Chinese medicine for this book came from the following sources:

Tierra, Dr. Michael. *Chinese Traditional Herbal Medicine Vol. 1: Diagnosis and Treatment.* Twin Lakes, WI: Lotus Press, 1998.

Kaptchuk, Ted J. *The Web That Has No Weaver.* Chicago: Congdon & Weed, 1983.

Reid, Daniel. *The Complete Book of Chinese Health and Healing: Guarding the Three Treasures.* Boston: Shambhala Publications, 1995.

INDEX BY AILMENT

Index by Action

Index by Latin Name

Index by Common Name

INDEX BY THAI NAME

GENERAL INDEX

Australian Bush Flower Essences
by Ian White

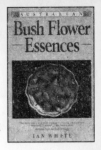

An informative yet personal picture of fifty bush flower essences as well as detailed information about their preparation and use in all areas of healing.

PUBLISHED BY FINDHORN PRESS • ISBN 0-905249-84-4

Bach Flower Remedies for Animals
by Helen Graham and Gregory Vlamis

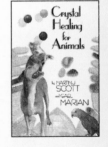

This books offers descriptions of each of the 38 Bach Flower Remedies, with their application in the treatment of a range of domestic animals, including horses. It also describes diagnostic symptoms, animal by animal, together with appropriate treatment regimes.

PUBLISHED BY FINDHORN PRESS • ISBN 1-899171-72-X

Crystal Healing for Animals
by Martin J Scott and Gael Mariani

Crystal healing is as effective and potent a healing art today as it was in the time of the ancient Egyptians. It is even more effective with animals than humans and any pet owner or animal caregiver can easily learn the basic techniques of choosing and cleansing crystals, , dowsing and crystal massage, making crystal essences, and the use of crystal layouts in healing.

PUBLISHED BY FINDHORN PRESS • ISBN 1-899171-24-X

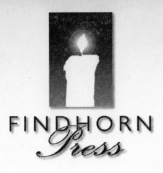

FINDHORN
Press

Findhorn Press is a publishing business of the Findhorn Community which has grown around the Findhorn Foundation in northern Scotland.

For further information about the Findhorn Foundation and the Findhorn Community, please contact:

Findhorn Foundation

The Visitors Centre
The Park, Findhorn IV36 3TY, Scotland, UK
tel 01309 690311• fax 01309 691301
email vcentre@findhorn.org
www.findhorn.org

For a complete Findhorn Press catalogue, please contact:

Findhorn Press

305a The Park, Findhorn

Forres IV36 3TE
Scotland, UK
Tel 01309 690582
freephone 0800-389-9395
Fax 01309 690036

If you live in the USA or Canada, please send your request to:

Findhorn Press

c/o Lantern Books
One Union Square West, Suite 201
New York, NY 10003-3303

Wherever you live, you can consult our catalogue online at

findhornpress.com

and email us at

info@findhornpress.com